# The Sweetest of All Inventions

By Lisa Clark

Australia

Copyright © 2023 by Lisa Clark.

All rights reserved. No part of this publication may be reproduced, distributed or transmitted in any form or by any means, including photocopying, recording, or other electronic or mechanical methods, without the prior written permission of the publisher, except in the case of brief quotations embodied in critical reviews and certain other noncommercial uses permitted by copyright law. For permission requests, write to the publisher, addressed "Attention: Permissions Coordinator," at the address below.

Lisa Clark c/- Intertype Publish and Print
Unit 45, 125 Highbury Road
BURWOOD VIC 3125
Australia
www.intertype.com.au

**Ordering Information:**
Quantity sales. Special discounts are available on quantity purchases by corporations, associations, and others. For details, contact the "Special Sales Department" at the address above.

The Sweetest of All Inventions/ Lisa Clark. —1st ed.
ISBN 978-0-6458106-2-2

**Disclaimers:**
This is a non-fiction memoir mostly written from the perspective of Lisa Harris (nee Clark). The events of the book are portrayed to the best of Lisa's memory and the memory of other people's perspectives featured throughout. These other contributors have also been credited accordingly. Whilst the memories and dialogue are not copied verbatim from the true word-for-word transcript of each conversation and event; they are written to represent the general feeling and meaning of what was said in each instance.

The author in no way represents or has the endorsement of the companies, corporations, or brands mentioned in this book.

The content of this book is for informational purposes only and is not intended to diagnose, treat, cure, or prevent any condition or disease. It does not substitute for the advice of a health professional.

# Contents

ACKNOWLEDGMENTS ................................................................. 9

STAN CLARK – FOREWORD .................................................... 11

A GENIUS IS BORN .................................................................... 17

A YOUNG MAN'S FUTURE ....................................................... 21

A PARTNERSHIP IS FORMED .................................................. 25

NEW LIFE JOURNEY ................................................................. 29

MY ARRIVAL BECOMES DAD'S DESTINY ........................... 33

STOLEN ........................................................................................ 37

UNWELCOME DIAGNOSIS ..................................................... 41

WORKSHOP UNDER THE HOUSE ........................................ 45

SCHOOL OF ELECTRONICS .................................................... 47

MY FIRST JOB ............................................................................. 49

LIVING WITH DIABETES ......................................................... 53

PARTY TIME ............................................................................... 57

EARLY MANAGEMENT ............................................................ 59

PHENOMENON IN THE MAKING ......................................... 61

LET'S MANUFACTURE THIS CREATION ............................. 65

NEW AND IMPROVED MODELS ............................................ 75

| | |
|---|---|
| OTHER INTERESTS | 77 |
| A GROWING BUSINESS | 79 |
| A PERFECT TEAM | 83 |
| FACTORY PROGRESSION | 87 |
| THE FACE OF THE BUSINESS | 91 |
| ANOTHER AUSTRALIAN FIRST | 95 |
| THE BEGINNING OF THE END | 99 |
| MY NEWFOUND ROLE | 103 |
| A NEW YET COMPLICATED BEGINNING | 107 |
| MY FIRST BORN | 113 |
| NEW DEVELOPMENT | 117 |
| CARD READING | 119 |
| PAPER MEETING | 121 |
| PREPARE FOR TAKEOFF | 125 |
| LAST VOCATION | 135 |
| THE PROPOSAL | 139 |
| TRAGIC DIAGNOSIS | 141 |
| A PERFECT WEDDING DAY | 145 |
| THE NEXT STAGE | 147 |
| WELCOME BUT CONCERNING NEWS | 149 |
| THE ANXIOUS ARRIVAL | 155 |

LOCATION CHANGE ............................................................. 157

THE NOT-SO-GREAT ESCAPE ............................................. 163

BUILT WITH LOVE ................................................................ 169

THE TOUGHEST DECISION ................................................. 173

SAYING GOODBYE TO A HERO........................................... 175

BUILDING NEW MEMORIES................................................. 179

EXEPTIONAL PROJECT ........................................................ 181

A LONG PAINFUL ROAD ...................................................... 183

A FABULOUS JOURNEY ....................................................... 189

*A tribute and special thanks to my Dad, Stanley Clark, for his amazing contribution to millions of diabetics around the world.*

*Dad may your legacy be recognized through future generations.*

# ACKNOWLEDGMENTS

The Author acknowledges the work and support of Diabetes Australia. Diabetes Australia is the national organisation supporting all people living with or at risk of diabetes, working in collaboration with member organisations, people with lived experience, health professionals, researchers and the community. 10% of authors profits from sales of THE SWEETEST OF ALL INVENTIONS will be donated to Diabetes Australia in recognition of the support provided to Stan Clark by the organisation and to support the vital work of Diabetes Australia to improve the lives of people living with or at risk of diabetes.

It is with my greatest thanks to the following people, all who have helped me achieve this very important tribute to my Dad Stan Clark. My gratitude for their contribution to my book is greatly appreciated. Thanks to my Husband Craig, my Daughter Madison, and my Son Mitchell. Most of all, I would like to thank my Mum, Audrey Clark, for her unwavering support for my Dad. Without Mum, Dad would not have been able to successfully achieve one of the greatest inventions in the history of diabetes.

I also give thanks and acknowledgement to Brendan Ford. Brendan is currently studying for a double degree in Law and Media, together with Communications (majoring in journalism and non-fiction writing). Brendan assisted with editing, altering, and making sure the book flowed correctly. Being a type 1 diabetic, Brendan also understood my need to get this untold story published.

* Diabetes Australia
* Emeritus Professor Martin Silink
* Professor Stephen Twigg
* Adjunct Associate Professor Margaret McGill
* ResMed
* Robert Styles
* Powerhouse Museum
* Hannah Rachael Photography
* Kevin Davis – Newspix
* Tim Perry
* Imogen Tear
* Intertype Publishing and Printing
* Literary contributors
* Friends and extended family

# STAN CLARK – FOREWORD

I met Lisa and her parents in 1975 at the diabetes clinic when she was 8 years old, some 3 years after she had been diagnosed with type 1 diabetes. At that time, I had been recently appointed to the Royal Alexandra Hospital for Children (RAHC) to develop a specialised department in paediatric diabetes and endocrinology.

In the 1970s, diabetes clinics were held weekly, and generally children would attend every 3 months. Each time the height and weight were carefully charted to make sure that the growth and development were as expected. A detailed history was taken of any issues, especially of diabetes control, and a general examination was undertaken. Diabetes control was assessed from a record of the twice daily urine tests measuring the amount of glucose excreted by the kidney, which indirectly indicated the blood glucose levels. The urine tests were either hated or accepted unwillingly since there were no other options at the time. The urine tests were made even more intrusive by testing the sample only after double voiding. The information from the urine testing guided changes to the dose of insulin (beef or pork), the length of action of the insulin preparation (short, medium or long-acting), as well as the number of daily injections.

In 1965 research had developed a new way to measure blood glucose levels that used a colorimetric method. A small drop of blood from a finger prick was placed on a strip. After 60 seconds the generated colour was then compared against a chart on the bottle for a semi-quantitative assessment of blood glucose. This early strip was only for physicians' offices, not for home use (1).

The principle behind the method employed ingenious chemistry. An enzyme (glucose oxidase) was embedded in the pad at the end of the strip.

Glucose oxidase acted on glucose in the drop of blood to create hydrogen peroxidase, which in turn was able to oxidise a chromogen to change its colour. The depth of the colour on the strip reflected the amount of hydrogen peroxidase produced, which in turn reflected the glucose level in the blood drop.

In 1970 a reflectance meter was developed to measure the depth of the colour on the stip. The principle of this was to use a beam of blue light of a known wavelength and measure how much of this light was reflected from the coloured pad. The depth of the colour read by the reflectance meter was then able to provide a more accurate measure of the blood glucose level.

At the time, reflectance meters were only sold to hospitals and laboratories. The meters were large, bulky, cumbersome (affectionately referred to as "the brick") and needed to be connected to a power point. The RAHC had a few of these and had started to use them at the bedside for immediate blood glucose results. They were expensive, to be used only by professionals, and completely unavailable outside the hospital system.

At this time in 1978, I attended a lecture from a visiting diabetes specialist from London. He presented the story of four pregnant women with type 1 diabetes, who had been admitted to hospital to monitor and control their diabetes. The treatment involved bed rest in hospital, diet and regular bedside blood testing and frequent insulin adjustments to keep glucose levels as close as possible to targets. The women, however, convinced their doctors that instead of being in hospital for the remainder of their pregnancy, they could do this just as well at home. Thus, they were sent home with a professional reflectance meter and strips. The result was that they were able to achieve similar results in their blood glucose levels at home as they had achieved in hospital. The social and emotional benefits of being at home with their families for the remainder of their pregnancy were immense. I was deeply impressed by this clinical presentation, which demonstrated that people with diabetes, when given the means and appropriate diabetes education, were able to measure their own blood glucose and use this information to fine-tune their own insulin treatment and improve their diabetes control.

Soon after hearing this presentation, Lisa had to come into hospital because her diabetes control was proving to be difficult and urine testing failed to provide sufficient information to allow changes to be made to her insulin treatment. In hospital, bedside glucose testing using strips and a reflectance meter started to reveal useful information, so I decided to send Lisa home for the weekend with "the brick" and strips, and to come back on Monday. They attended the hospital on the following Monday and returned the hospital's reflectance meter, saying that I could have it back. I enquired whether home blood glucose monitoring was not for them. They smiled and Stan quietly indicated that he had worked out how it functioned and had made their own meter over the weekend. I was astounded and then excited at the possibility of providing this to the other children in the diabetes clinic.

After confirming the accuracy of Stan's reflectance meter in reading the strips, I enquired whether he could make more. The reply was an enthusiastic "yes". I was then able to convince the Board of Management of the Hospital of the benefits of home blood glucose monitoring in improving diabetes control in the children attending the diabetes clinic. The Board agreed to advance $6000 to allow the manufacture of the instruments (named the RAHC Glucose Tester) and by the end of the year most of the children in the clinic were using Stan's machine. To my knowledge, the RAHC diabetes clinic was one of the first centres to pioneer home blood glucose monitoring in children with type 1 diabetes. This was only made possible by Stan's vision, knowledge and leadership in bringing affordable blood glucose monitoring out of the hospitals and into the community.

Pilot studies in the UK and the USA in 1978 using the cumbersome professional reflectance meters demonstrated that adults with type 1 diabetes could monitor their own blood glucose and use this information to adjust their own insulin therapy and improve their diabetes control (2,3). Importantly, these studies also demonstrated that patient satisfaction was improved. The authors of these studies predicted the need for smaller blood glucose reflectance meters to be made available, but no one, not even the large pharmaceutical industries, were manufacturing convenient affordable reflectance meters at the time. Very few understood the hunger in people with diabetes for a tool which gave them knowledge and some agency in managing their diabetes, which often seemed to be unpredictable. Stan understood the urgency and he acted years ahead of industry. He made it possible for small, portable reflectance meters to be made available to people with diabetes for use in the home. He gave them hope. For the first time for many, diabetes control started to make sense and became possible.

To put this into perspective: Were there any hurdles along the way? The answer is yes. The concept of patients being empowered to adjust their insulin doses based on self-monitoring was regarded by many in the health profession as potentially dangerous. Concerns were expressed that a child would not be able to cope with the pain and not understand why their parents needed to prick their finger several times a day. It was thought that I should not promote, what was deemed by some, an unethical treatment. Many an adult with diabetes, struggling with the psychological hurdle of pricking their own finger several times a day, was cajoled into home blood glucose monitoring by the example of a three-year-old bravely and calmly putting their finger forward for a finger prick.

With the provision of appropriate support and access to diabetes education, home blood glucose monitoring empowered people with diabetes to improve and intensify their diabetes control by self-adjusting insulin doses. Pioneering Diabetes Educators like Marg McGill developed multidisciplinary "diabetes teams" to impart essential knowledge and skills to people with diabetes, that enabled them to understand and best use the information gained from their home blood glucose monitoring.

In the 1980s essential questions focussed on how close to normal the targets of intensified diabetes control should be and whether the chronic complications of diabetes (including retinopathy, renal failure, neuropathy and cardiovascular disease) could be prevented or ameliorated by better diabetes control. The answers to these questions only became possible following the development of the Glycosylated Haemoglobin or HbA1c test (a measure of how much glucose had linked to haemoglobin over the previous 3 months) (4-6). By using home blood glucose monitoring and HbA1c testing, the Diabetes Control and Complications Trial (DCCT) demonstrated the overwhelming benefits of intensive therapy over conventional therapy in preventing chronic diabetic complications as well as in decreasing the risks of hypoglycaemia (7).

Home blood glucose monitoring is undoubtedly one of the most important therapeutic developments in intensifying diabetes control. It is hard to underestimate the effect of home blood glucose monitoring on the lives on people with type 1 diabetes. On a day-to-day basis, home blood glucose monitoring led to immense improvements in their quality of life, and in the long-term, it gave people with type 1 diabetes the power over the inevitability of developing chronic complications. Stan Clark and his portable and affordable reflectance meters made it possible for blood glucose monitoring to move out of hospitals, into the community and into the home. For this, to thousands of people with diabetes, Stan was truly a hero.

Martin Silink

Martin Silink AO MB BS (Hons 1, USyd) MD FRACP
Emeritus Professor of Medicine, University of Sydney
Honorary President, International Diabetes Federation (IDF)
Past President, International Society of Pediatric and Adolescent Diabetes (ISPAD)
Past President, Australasian Paediatric Endocrine Group (APEG)

References:
1. Hirsch IB. Introduction: History of Glucose Monitoring. In: Role of Continuous Glucose Monitoring in Diabetes Treatment. Arlington (VA): American Diabetes Association; 2018 Aug. PMID: 34251770 Bookshelf ID: NBK538968 DOI: 10.2337/db20181-1
2. Sönksen PH, Judd SL, Lowy C. Home monitoring of blood-glucose. Method for improving diabetic control. Lancet 1978;1:729-732
3. Walford S, Gale EA, Allison SP, Tattersall RB. Self-monitoring of blood-glucose. Improvement of diabetic control. Lancet 1978;1:732-745
4. Rahbar S. An abnormal hemoglobin in red cells of diabetics. Clin Chim Acta 1968;22:296–8

5. Gabbay KH. Glycosylated hemoglobin and diabetic control. N Engl J Med 1976;295:443–4
6. Trivelli LA, Ranney HM, Lai HT. Hemoglobin components in patients with diabetes mellitus. N Engl J Med 1971;7:353–7
7. The Diabetes Control and Complications Trial Research Group. The Effect of Intensive Treatment of Diabetes on the Development and Progression of Long-Term Complications in Insulin-Dependent Diabetes Mellitus. N Engl J Med 1993; 29:977-9

CHAPTER 1

# A GENIUS IS BORN

My Dad, Stanley Clark, was born in Sheffield, Yorkshire, England on the 16th April 1934.

Sheffield is a city in the English county of South Yorkshire. It gained international reputation for steel production in the 19th century and its population boomed during the Industrial Revolution. Innovations developed throughout – including the famous Sheffield Steel giving the name "Steel City" to Sheffield. It is also known for its beautiful, picturesque scenery. Famous singer Joe Cocker was even born in the city and titled one of his albums "Sheffield Steel".

My Dad was born to Lily Clark (nee Palmer) and Charles Clark. He was the youngest son of six children although, sadly, there were originally eight children. Two of his brothers died incredibly young and although they passed away separately – both within a noticeably short time frame.

Dad was the second youngest child. He had three sisters and two remaining brothers.

Charlie was my Dad's eldest brother. He was born in May 1920, followed by a sister Lilly in February 1922. Wilfred was born in October 1924 and Harry was born in November 1925. Wilfred died at two-and-a-half and Harry died at the age of one. Grandad and Grandma then went on to have more children. Ron was born in September 1927, followed by Ada in 1929. My grandparents were then blessed with my Dad in 1934. Dad and his brothers and sisters then welcomed another baby sister, June, born in June 1935.

My Dad was always the favourite of the family. He never complained, never sulked, never had a bad word to say about anyone. His entire family loved him, and he was, from what my cousins have told me, the favourite child and much-loved brother to both his sisters and brothers.

Dad grew up during the Second World War and was greatly influenced by his father. From a young age, my Grandad studied astronomy, photography and then became interested in the then-new "radio". Grandad was privileged to have lived at the time of John Logie Baird and knew of his experiments including the mechanical and electronic television.

In the early 1920's, Grandad, Charles, worked in England as an engineer at Dorman Long. They were an engineering consultancy and equipment manufacturer for the construction of long-span bridges, power stations, refineries, and other large building structures. Notably, the company built the Sydney Harbour Bridge. With young children, this would have been a lucrative job for Grandad.

In 1924, Dorman Long were granted the contract to build the Sydney Harbour Bridge and my Grandad was asked to be one of the team to move their families to Australia and build it. I do not know a great deal of first-hand information about my Grandad, but I must say that if he was anything like my Dad, Grandad was selected for the job based on his knowledge, his ability, his workmanship, and his work ethic. He must have been very well respected by Dorman Long to be offered such a fantastic opportunity.

As my Grandad and Grandma had young children, it was my Grandma's decision to halt Grandad's opportunity and offer. She was concerned about the consequences an overseas move would have on the kid's upbringing. Also, she was extremely close to her Dad and refused to leave him.

I can understand her anxieties. In those days, it was all boat travel and the thought of sea sickness with young children for weeks on end would have certainly put me off the same idea – especially as the majority of boats that travelled from England to Australia were extremely limited with stabilizers. If my Grandma was as close to her Dad as I with mine, then I would have made the exact same decision.

Grandad stayed with Dorman Long for many years. He continued to work there during the great depression, and for many years after. He then decided to buy himself a lorry (truck) and drove it for many years both before and during his retirement.

Grandad told my Dad fascinating true stories about astronomy as well as radio and how it worked. He also spoke to Dad about television and a host of other fantastic and fascinating things, including morse code.

He mentioned to Dad that he had seen Halley's Comet and mentioned that it would be around again at the time my Dad would become a man. He asked Dad to promise to look for it when the time came and sure enough, Dad was lucky enough to see Halley's Comet from his bed in 1986. Dad remembered the promise he had made, and thankfully was able to keep. Mum and Dad, at the time, owned a house across the road from Warriewood Blow Hole on Sydney's Northern beaches. The view over the water was the perfect view for Dad to see the comet.

Growing up, electronics was my Dad's favourite hobby. My eldest cousin on his side of the family, Geoff, has informed me that he remembers his uncle Stan always creating electronic things. He was always showing Geoff how things worked and was always producing new creations.

Grandad always encouraged him to make things out of old parts from a shop that they used to go to in Sheffield called Bardwell's. This was an electronics super store which was originally a TV and radio repair shop. It first opened in the 1940's and as the years went on, it expanded to sell any electronic component that was known to man. Unfortunately, it closed only a few years ago after 70 years of operation as a family business.

Dad and Grandad made things such as shocking coils, crystal sets, telephones, and telescopes – all of which were put together with sealing wax, string, and cardboard. Dad said they used to experiment with anything that was easy to access from Bardwell's.

The war ended in 1945 and lucky for Dad, vast amounts of electronic, radio, radar and scientific equipment became available on the war surplus market. Dad would do odd jobs to save the money which enabled him to go to Bardwell's in Sheffield and buy the wonderful ex-surplus gear.

Dad made one and two valve radios using large 1920 and 1930 valves. He would tell me that as a little boy he would love to bike ride. As he got older and able to venture alone, he would ride for hours by himself. Dad used to dream of being able to listen to a radio while he was riding his bicycle, so he made a radio in the form of a tube (like a thick bicycle tyre pump) which he taped to the crossbar. With this he could listen with his earphones to the radio as he travelled around town. He often told me, many years later, it would have been the first Walkman.

I can imagine it was during these rides he was thinking about many electronic creations. It was during his teenage years – filled with many hours riding around town – that he became interested in miniaturisation and of course the magic of television.

At this stage, Grandad undoubtedly had absolutely no idea that these events would lead his youngest son to create a worldwide phenomenon many years later.

Throughout these teenage years, Dad was always a bit of a loaner but had a great friend called Jimmy Barnes! Yes, you would ask if this was the Cold Chisel lead singer – but although Jimmy was a great man – he was not the Jimmy Barnes that most would think!

Jimmy was a great friend to my Dad for decades until he sadly died in his later years. I can imagine that Dad spent many hours with Jimmy showing him how to pull things apart and make something else using the same parts. Although Jimmy was not electronically inclined, the way my Dad would explain how something worked was nothing short of miraculous, yet simple – a true sign of genius.

My Dad's talent, and later ability, is what my story is about. My story will leave you, the reader, enlightened, amazed, and totally gobsmacked by the love, the determination, the knowledge, and inspiring success that my Dad achieved. This story is about Dad's invention of a worldwide phenomenon which was created by his love for me, his only child.

CHAPTER 2

# A YOUNG MAN'S FUTURE

As Dad became a young man, he had jobs that always involved electronics, magnets, and various other projects. He worked on anything technical, and anything that had some kind of mystery with how it worked.

In May 1950, my Dad went to work for a business called Jessop Saville and Company Ltd – a Sheffield-based steel organization – after working for a company of electric motor repairers and armature winders. At that stage he was already studying for his Ordinary National Certificate in Electrical Engineering, and it was at Jessop Saville where he started work in the Magnetic Research Laboratory. His duties consisted of the testing of magnetic alloys which involved a considerable amount of instrumental work.

In September 1952, at the age of eighteen, Dad was conscripted into the National Service which was a requirement at that time. He always had a keen interest in aeronautics and therefore chose to enter the Royal Air Force – or the RAF as he used to tell me as a little girl. He was deployed to Checkpoint Charlie in Berlin, otherwise known as Checkpoint C. Dad was trained during his time in the RAF in radio direction finding and mobile communications. This was an absolute dream for my Dad as he always had that keen interest in radio's, TV's, together with anything regarding communication and technology.

He spoke with me about one specific incident where he was on night duty and heard rustling noises outside his station tent. Given this was of great concern to him, he promptly shouted out "I've got a gun" and with trepidation he walked forward towards the opening of the tent. He was confronted with a man's hand, a large and bejewelled ring on each finger, pulling the flap of the tent aside. The man in question raised his hands in surrender, seeing Dad with his rifle pointed in his direction. As it turned out, the man had just escaped from East Germany and just wanted asylum in West Germany.

Dad had many stories to tell about his post World War II time in Berlin as a National Serviceman and was immensely proud of his time in the RAF. One thing Dad taught me about his time in the Air Force was how to polish shoes properly! As I grew up and learnt the art of perfect shoe polishing, I was always proud to go to school with the most perfectly shiny shoes.

After Dad's time in the RAF, he returned to Jessop Saville. On his return, he went back into the Magnetic Research Department, but his role then was workshop duties involving instrument repairs, coil winding, and all aspects of instrument technology in relation to magnetic testing. He was respected for his great initiative and a distinct flair for instrument design and repair to such an extent that Dad's duties were extended to cover research and development work for any section of the company's research department. He was tasked with all the developmental work of electrical equipment.

Dad worked on projects such as the design of equipment for the stirring of molten steel during continuous casting. He developed certain electronic safety devices in connection with gamma-ray inspection and he also designed and built magnetic crack detecting equipment for steel inspection. Dad then progressed to the electronics section of Jessop Saville's research department. His duties included the maintenance and servicing of ultrasonic equipment, high sensitivity electronic temperature controllers, instrumentation in connection with spectrographic analysis.

During his time with Jessop-Saville Dad completed his Course for the Ordinary National Certificate in Electrical Engineering and he also became a member of the Institution of Electronics. Dad did not serve a recognised apprenticeship with Jessop-Saville simply because there was no apprenticeship scheme in operation that would have given the required adequate training in electronics. He was beyond any training that an apprenticeship offered. Dad therefore obtained additional training by part-time study and by working under the direct supervision of graduates and qualified personnel with extensive experience in electronics.

It was during his time at Jessop-Saville Limited that Dad met my Mum. My Mum worked in administration answering the phone and taking mail around the building's offices. Shortly after, she got promoted to a position in the Bloom Grinders Department (which is the surface conditioning of steel) and only a few months later she was promoted again to the cashier's office into their wages and accounts section.

My Mum, Audrey Limb, was the middle child of William and Winifred Limb. She was born 24th October 1937 in Sheffield, Yorkshire, England. Mum had an older sister, Joyce and a younger brother, John. Mum also grew up in Sheffield. My Mum was a stunning young woman who had the most adorable dimples in her cheeks. She was far from shy as her personality was always happy, friendly, and simply someone my Dad could not resist. Dad was an incredibly quiet person and was reasonably shy, so it took some time before he was confident enough to ask Mum out. From what Mum has told me Dad would go to collect his pay from her and they would talk for ages about anything and everything.

Jessop-Saville Limited held a dance every now and then in City Hall Sheffield, Mum had the job of selling tickets for the dance and it was at the City Hall dance that my Dad finally picked up the courage to ask my Mum to dance with him.

Mum and Dad would often laugh at some of the stories of their courtship. Even 60 years later, my Mum still laughs about Dad taking her on a motor bike. It was the middle of winter, and the English winter is freezing cold and certainly not a trip most people would consider on a motor bike at that time of year. With jackets, boots and helmets Dad gets prepared to take Mum on a bike ride so she could experience his new motor bike. The bike, a classic BSA was not brand new, as Dad preferred to spend his money on electronic parts rather than spend a large amount of money on something new that would, over time, lose value. It was new to him as he had always wanted a motor bike so the thrill of having one of his own was a whole new experience. Once they were both on the bike and had travelled a brief time without any hiccups, Dad came to a street which required him to make a 90-degree right hand turn.

Mum had never been on a motor bike prior to this so she had it in her mind that she needed to lean the opposite way to Dad to keep the bike upright! Thankfully, Dad was able to keep the motor bike from falling over and with a streak of luck neither of them fell off, thankfully, as I possibly wouldn't be here to tell the story.

After the shock had left the two of them, Dad decided to ride his motor bike solo from that time on. Mum was extremely happy with this as when she attempted to get off the bike, after their thrill-seeking experience, her knees were frozen bent. It took ages for them to straighten and thaw out.

CHAPTER 3

# A PARTNERSHIP IS FORMED

Mum and Dad married on 30th March 1957 in Sheffield. Their wedding was in a beautiful old English stone church landscaped by the sunlight of a beautiful day. Mum carried a bouquet of flowers which were of a soft tangerine colour.

They moved into their own home, which was comfortable for them both and, of course, Dad was able to create a suitable working space for his electronic creations. He had always, prior to getting married, tinkered on a daily basis with electronics, Dad would go into his work area after dinner and create some of the most mind-blowing gadgets using his vast electronics knowledge. He worked electronics, he slept electronics. It was his hobby and passion. Dad, at the age of twenty-three, made Mum a miniature television which I imagine would be the first portable television. Dad had lovingly made this for my Mum as a wedding present. It had a two and three-quarter inch screen and cost him approximately 12 English pounds. It was made of nineteen tiny valves and the aerial was a 3 ft piece of wire. It received both ITV and BBC transmission and it ran from mains power or a car battery. Today, this miniature television is in the Television and Photographic Museum in Bradford, England. It is displayed next to the Original World First Prototype of the John Logie Baird television. His creation of a miniature TV is what my Dad was about. He was brilliant and was always thinking of something to make and from this brilliance, his next creation was utterly remarkable.

Dad, at this stage, had started his own TV repair business and repaired TV's and record players after work. Both Mum and Dad continued to work for Jessop-Saville until December 1958 and due to the repair business going crazy with work, they decided to both leave Jessop-Saville and open a shop of their own. They worked together, Dad repairing TV's, radio's, record players etc. Mum would help however she could, but she also spent much of her time in the shop selling products that were electronic, as they had made the decision to sell electrical items and small goods such as kettles.

The shop was on the main street of Attercliffe Common, situated on the main road that went through the high street of Sheffield. There were many different shops along the road including a wool shop. The shops were close to the road and had a large picture window and a room at the front which is where the tenants of each shop would display their products. During summer, the heat would come through the front glass window and keep the shops at a beautiful temperature. Each shop was approximately twenty square metres however the space was reasonably square in layout. There was a small dividing wall which led to the little kitchenette which housed a ridiculously small sink, a cold-water tap, together with a small bench with a little cupboard underneath. There was only a very small space behind the dividing wall for the storage of Dad's electronic parts however they made do with the space they felt lucky to have. The toilet was quite a walk to the end of the shops and around the back, up a very narrow cobblestoned pathway to a single toilet with a small sink. Mum always said that she hated needing to go to the toilet in winter when she was at the shop, as English winters were often literally freezing and a trip to the toilet was like a punishment.

My Mum had a fascination for music. She knew a great beat when she heard one and with several people coming in to either buy a new record player or repair anyone's old record player, Mum decided she would contact a company in London and ask them if she could sell their records in the shop. It works out she had to lodge an application to be granted permission to sell records. The big boss turned up from the record company, he came from London, and with my Mum's undeniable charm and initiative, he granted her the application she required.

THE SWEETEST OF ALL INVENTIONS • 27

Within months, Mum had many of the latest records by several hit artists at the time. She always had stock of all the popular records which were requested by her customers. She had all the latest Beatles records and as I was growing up, she would sing a song to me "My Old Man's a Dustman". This was a hit record by Lonnie Donegan.

Mum and Dad owned a highly successful small business in Sheffield and within a few years Mum got hungry for another adventure and challenge. They noticed a shop across the road from their existing shop had become vacant so decided to open a "Pea and Pie" shop. Pies in the 1950's were a simple meat pie, certainly nothing like the pies today made of curry chicken, satay chicken, beef, and mushroom, any flavour of pie you can imagine these days.

Mum would collect the pies from a bakery in Sheffield at 6am every morning and take them back to their shop where she would start the ovens and later load the pies into the then warm ovens. She would soak the dried marrowfat peas overnight in baking soda, so they were ready for the pies the following morning. They had a roaring business and they both worked very long hours but absolutely loved what both shops offered and rewarded them with.

Mum tells me about the people that would visit both shops and they built up a great rapport with the local customers and other shop owners. Mum had a time where her peas had failed. She arrived at the shop one cold and snowy morning, unlocked the shop, and began her day as she did every other morning. She would always put the ovens on as soon as she arrived and prepared the rest of the shop for her busy lunch time rush. This one morning, her heart sank as she opened the pan to the peas. The peas had gone rock hard. Her usual mushy peas were certainly not mushy on this particular day, and she was in a state of confusion as to why the peas had not worked! She decided to speak with her neighbours in the fish and chip shop. The people in the chip shop felt sorry for her so they decided to give her some of their mushy peas which would certainly help her out for that day. Thankfully, due to their kind generosity, she was able to supply all her customers with her pies and peas, as she did every other day.

Mum would give any food leftovers from each day to the less fortunate people that were homeless. Three people she often told me about when I was a little girl, and she still remembers to this day, were her regulars looking for a meal. Their nicknames were Duke of Darnell, Herman the German, and Vinegar Lil. Mum made these names up for them after regular conversations and getting to know them personally. All the people that Mum knew whether homeless, well to do, or simply the locals, loved her, cared for her, they would all move mountains for her. This particularly put Dad's mind at rest as although he was never far away with having both shops close to each other, he knew that Mum had someone always looking out for her if needed.

In 1963, Dad was offered some work with a company called Marrison & Catherall Ltd. This was a company heavily involved in magnets. During Dad's time with them he designed the first 30 volt, 1000-amp DC heat treatment unit for use in "Packaged Magnetron Magnets". This was the first ever used in Europe and the world. Its use enabled the magnets to be cast in one piece which therefore allowed a smaller more efficient unit. This left Mum with the task of running both shops all by herself. Thankfully, as they were across the road from each other she would run backwards and forwards to each shop so Dad could continue his work at Marrison and Catherall Ltd. Dad then went back to the repair shop after work to repair the items that people had brought into the TV repair shop during that day.

Mum and Dad continued with great success in both their shops for about five years and then Dad had an idea that stemmed from his parents not taking the opportunity to move to Sydney, Australia. He mentioned it to Mum and although Mum was still young and did not want to leave her family, she did not want to take away from Dad a similar possibility that was offered to my Grandad 40 odd years earlier.

# CHAPTER 4

# NEW LIFE JOURNEY

With Australia in desperate need for immigrants who possessed technical skills, it was in 1964 that Mum and Dad left their home in Sheffield, their business's, their family, and their friends, and sailed as 10-pound poms from Southampton on a ship called the Aurelia. The Aurelia was launched in December 1938 in Hamburg. The boat was used for fifty-eight first class passengers in the luxuriously appointed amidship superstructure. In 1940, it was taken over by the German Navy and converted into a submarine/U-boat depot. During the war, the Aurelia became a submarine repair ship, spending much of her time in Norway. The ship was finally captured by the British in 1945. It was the British who refitted the ship to eventually carry passengers, taking Mum and Dad on their new adventure through the Mediterranean and the Suez Canal to Perth. They then sailed on from Perth to Sydney. My Mum was extremely seasick during the entire trip, and although she was always very slim, she lost a lot more weight during the journey.

After a torturous time at sea, Mum and Dad arrived in Sydney and were transported to a house in Arncliffe, a suburb approximately eleven kilometres south of Sydney's CBD. They moved into a lady's flat above her house – a house where the lady was looking after two young boys that were not her own. The lady was not married and from what Mum understood, she had taken the boys under her wing to care for them. The reason she was looking after the boys is not information the lady offered and Mum, therefore, did not feel it was her duty to ask how the boys came into her care. From what Mum knew they were two young brothers.

Mum struggled to settle into the small flat above the house as her and Dad had left a beautiful home in England and the flat was old and slightly run down. Mum and Dad's bathroom in their old home was exceptionally clean and was inside their home. The flat did not have its own bathroom. It was down a set of outside stairs and was at the end of the garden. The bath and toilet were in separate rooms and were shared both with Mum and Dad together with the lady and the two boys.

In May 1964 Dad was offered a job with a company called Thomas Electronics of Australia Pty Ltd as a Senior Electronics Technician. Dad was responsible for the correct operation of all processing and testing involving electronic equipment and circuitry. His duties included the design and supervision of manufacturing, together with the installation and testing of new equipment. He was also involved with items such as TV's sweep synchronisation generators, RF Power Oscillators, and conveyor activation equipment for TV tube cathode processing.

Dad, together with the help of an additional technician, was responsible for routine testing and periodic maintenance of all electronic equipment in the plant. This equipment included TV Picture Tube Testers, TV Receiver Chassis for life testing, 6 KW RF Power Generators, Ionisation Vacuum Gauge units, Thyratron Welding Timers and various process control equipment involving timers, oscillators, HV supplies.

Dad left Thomas Electronics in December 1966 and after a couple of weeks off during the Christmas break, he was offered a job with the Department of Motor Transport. His position was a Grade 1 Engineering Assistant. This involved repairs and manufacturing of the street cameras in Sydney city. Dad stayed with the Department of Motor Transport for several years.

Shortly before Dad left Thomas Electronics, Mum and Dad decided to purchase their own home. They decided to settle on Sydney's Northern Beaches in Wheeler Heights and purchased a block of land on which they had a three bedroom home built. Both Mum and Dad continued to commute to their jobs and thoroughly enjoyed returning to their new home every evening.

Towards the end of 1966, Mum was constantly sick. After several trips to the doctor, Mum found out she was pregnant. Mum and Dad had waited ten long years for the exciting news of having a baby however my poor Mum was sick during her entire pregnancy. Most of the way through, all she could eat was green apples without being sick. She suffered horrific morning sickness and for months, struggled to get through every day. There was already little weight on my Mum as she had always been slim, so for her to only be able to keep green apples down meant she was quite healthy, however at the end of her pregnancy she was extremely underweight.

CHAPTER 5

# MY ARRIVAL BECOMES DAD'S DESTINY

I was born in June 1967 in Crown Street Women's Hospital, Sydney. Thankfully without any problems due to Mum only being able to eat those green apples. This was during the time Dad was working for the Department of Motor Transport, so poor Dad was busy not only with work but also travelling from work to the hospital then home to Wheeler Heights.

The long working days for Dad was fine until Mum was told she could possibly have breast cancer. They found the lump shortly after I was born and Dad being the doting new father was determined to take me home to look after me. It works out that a long-time friend of Mum's was prepared to take the pressure off Dad and offered to take care of me until Mum was well enough to be able to come home. Dad collected me from the hospital in a wooden drawer and as I was born early, combined with Mum and Dad's long work hours they had not had the time to buy the baby items they so desperately needed. My Dad could always find a suitable option for just about anything he required so the wooden drawer became my cosy bassinet from the hospital to my temporary home.

I was welcomed with a fancy bassinet and some incredibly special people to take care of me. They spent many sleepless nights attending to me as a newborn baby. They had children of their own, all of which had grown up by the time I was brought into their home. Thankfully, several weeks later Mum was given the all-clear and the breast cancer tests returned a negative result, so I was able to be returned to my grateful, relieved Mum.

After my birth, Dad continued to work for the Department of Motor Transport however he had always been interested in tools and had always spent a reasonable amount of his wages saving for tools that were of good quality. Dad was in his elements when he was offered a job with Wolf Tools in January 1971. Wolf Tools was the best of the best for tools during the 1960's. It was a European brand that offered a wide range of high-quality power tools for the home handyman.

I remember my Dad having a company car with Wolf Tools. It was a posh car to me, and I thought my Dad was very important having that company car. I was too young to know what make of car it was, but I do clearly remember the car had brown leather seats and it had gold paintwork. It did have a boot, so I do remember Dad telling me it was called a sedan.

Dad spent many years at Wolf Tools which, for me meant many years of us driving around in luxury in the gold-coloured car with the most comfortable leather seats. I remember it having a very large glove box cause Dad would put his packed lunch in there that Mum would make for him every workday.

Dad was then offered a job with Hanimex in Brookvale, Sydney's Northern Beaches. This was a company that imported and distributed cameras, lenses and other photographic equipment in Australia and New Zealand. This would have created great memories for Dad as it would have taken him back to the days when his father taught him how to make telescopes out of cardboard. The company also distributed consumer electronics together with other non-photographic equipment and Dad was made their Technical Production Co-ordinator. He worked as an engineer in product development and provided technical assistance for manufacturing, it was at Hanimex that Dad met a man called Bob Styles. Bob and Dad became great friends, and it would be the start of a new friendship that would last for many years to come and the stories of their work and friendship continued throughout their careers.

When I was three years old, my Dad made me an electric car. I remember it had a canopy with pink tassels on it. Mum had obviously found the tassels at a haberdashery shop. It had a foot pedal which would move the car when I put my foot down. I would stop it by taking my foot off the foot pedal. Dad made it with a storage boot, just like his sedan that he had in his work at Wolf Tools, so I would pretend to be the milk man, the bread man, the ice cream man, although this was difficult in the hot summer due to the ice cream melting. If this were today, I would be known as the milk, bread, and ice cream person.

My Dad was constantly making me gadgets in his workshop. I remember a soap display that he made for me with lights. I also had a collection of fancy soaps which I would display on my dressing table. Dad got clear coloured pieces of Perspex and put battery operated lights in them. I had the most magnificent display for my soap collection. He then made me an upgraded model by making it out of clear, blue Perspex. My soap display most certainly then had pizzaz!

CHAPTER 6

# STOLEN

Early one morning, Mum and Dad woke up to find that Mum's car had been stolen from our driveway. It was in the very early hours of the morning, and it was carried out very quietly. Our driveway was not an easy driveway to contend with, let alone reverse in or out of with ease. We went to Dee Why Police Station to report it and after a few days, Dad was contacted and asked if we could go to Chatswood Police Station to file a more detailed report of the theft. The car was not to be found anywhere and although there was an intense search for the car, nothing showed up for months. My Mum knew her car down to a tee and even viewed from a distance she would know if it was or was not her car. It was a white 1962 Vauxhall Victor and Mum was heartbroken as she absolutely loved her car.

Mums work was having a Christmas party which was going to be held at night so with Dad being away at that time, she asked our neighbour to look after me for the night. I called her Aunty Josie, and I would spend time with her when Mum had to work, or Dad was not home. Aunty Josie loved me being with her and Mum knew that whenever I was with her, I was loved and cared for totally.

Mum left for the party, and it was about a one-hour drive away from where we lived. My Mum was dressed beautifully and, as always, looked stunning. The sun was about to set and just before she reached her destination, she saw her car... her stolen car... parked at a bus stop near Ryde in Sydney. Her heart missed a beat and she very quickly turned around and went back to see if it was her car. She had not had a great chance to look when she drove past the first time as it took her by surprise. Also, driving at the time, she did not want to take her eyes off the road to inspect it and cause an accident. After driving up to the car she knew that there was no one it. She stopped, got out of Dad's car, and immediately knew that the car in the bus stop was her Vauxhall Victor. Although the number plate was different, she still knew it was her car because of its idiosyncrasies. She knew she had to think quickly, and she also knew she did not want to leave the car unattended. She was aware that the bonnet had never locked properly so she could lift the bonnet without having to release the button inside the car to open it. All dressed up with her beautiful party dress on, she lifted the bonnet, disconnected the battery, and removed a spark plug lead which would stop the car from starting.

Thankfully, Mum's dress wasn't covered in grease, but she certainly needed to make sure that her car wasn't going anywhere. She drove Dad's car to the nearest petrol station and called the police. She had the direct number of the people she had been dealing with at Chatswood so thankfully she was able to speak with the appropriate people immediately, without having to tell them the full story. She also contacted my Dad's good friend, Barry, who was also my Godfather. He immediately left his house in Moorebank, near Bankstown, and drove directly to where Mum said she had spotted the car. Mum then left the petrol station and went back to the car. She then stood guarding her stolen car and waited for the police and Barry to arrive. While she was waiting, a man in another car stopped, got out of the car that he was a passenger in and approached Mum. He asked my Mum what she was doing with "his" car, so my Mum questioned him by saying "your" car. She said, "this is my car, and you stole it from my house." He began to argue with her, so she interrupted him and said, "I know your name and the police are on their way". Mum and Dad had been informed that the person in question was the head of a car stealing syndicate. Within a minute or two of Mum telling him that she knew everything about him, the police arrived and escorted him to the police station. Barry arrived just as the police took the man in question away. He made sure Mum was OK and was glad that Mum had finally, after months, found her car.

Mum left for her party, feeling very happy and proud of herself and continued her night with a big story to tell. The police also arranged for the car to be towed back to the police compound and be checked for fingerprints. Within a short period of time, Mum was able to collect her car and the only thing that was any different to when Mum had it initially, the number plate was a new one.

Dad arrived home absolutely amazed at my fabulous Mum for cracking a car stealing syndicate, although he was not happy with her for taking the possible risk of putting herself in real danger. After all, this man was wanted by the police.

CHAPTER 7

# UNWELCOME DIAGNOSIS

It was June 1972, and it was my fifth birthday. I was having a birthday party and my Mum always made me the best birthday cakes ever. For this birthday, Mum made me the most creative and colourful birthday cake I had ever seen. It was a "Hansel & Gretel" house. It was covered with freckles and chocolate stick biscuits. It also had pink musk sticks as the door frame and Mum used smarties and a variety of lollies that were popular in 1972!

I remember feeling slightly unwell before my friends were due to arrive however the excitement of my party was so overwhelming that I put that feeling aside and all thought of sickness seemed to just pale into insignificance. All my friends arrived and as it was winter, we spent my birthday party playing pass the parcel, hide & seek and pin the tail on the donkey. We also danced to all the music hits of 1972. Yes, at the age of five, I did have male friends that came to my party. Yes, even the boys were dancing!

During the party we had party pies, sausage rolls, fairy bread and lemonade. The party food just kept on coming and when the time came for me to cut the cake, I felt terrible. I did not have the heart to tell my Mum or my Dad as they had worked so hard to create a birthday party and a cake to remember. The time came for me to cut my magnificent cake. As my friends gathered around the table with the cake on it, they started to sing "Happy

Birthday to you". By the end of the cake cutting part of the party, I was seriously ready to sit down, be sick and go to sleep!

After all my friends had left, I continued having fun playing with my birthday gifts. Although I felt terrible, I simply thought that I was just tired and not only had too much excitement but also way too much to eat. The day had come to an end, and it was time for bed.

It was at this time that I always needed to go to the toilet. I would get up through the night, wake up either my Mum or my Dad because at the tender age of five, although I thought I was so grown up, a trip to the toilet in the cold of winter, was quite a daunting task. I started to do this several times a night, every night. I remember an incredible thirst so I would go to the bathroom, turn the cold tap on and drink for minutes at a time. This continued for weeks until my Dad, whose parents both were diagnosed with diabetes in later life, noticed the symptoms of diabetes.

After several visits to the local doctor, my Dad was stunned as the doctor told him that his suspicions were wrong and that the symptoms did not correlate with the common symptoms of diabetes. After yet another doctor's appointment elsewhere, it was suggested that Mum and Dad take me to have some blood tests and a glucose tolerance test to see what was wrong with me.

I clearly remember the place we went to in Dee Why which was not too far from our home. It was a shop that had been converted into a few rooms where they took blood from your arm. It was a pathology clinic, but I will always remember it as the place they took blood from your arm and made you drink horrible, sweet syrup. Obviously, not a great memory. These horrible blood tests were a very clear start to many more to come. After several hours of drinking sickly sweet syrup, followed with lots of blood tests, Mum and Dad were given the news that their 5-year-old, only child, was diagnosed with diabetes. My Dad's suspicions were extremely valid, especially after he watched his parents suffer with a disorder that would eventually take their lives due to diabetic complications. Dad's Mum was diagnosed with diabetes when Dad was ten years old and his Dad was diagnosed shortly after my grandmother.

A memory that I will always have is one of the nurses that took my blood had promised me that if I were brave and strong, she would make me something very special. My goodness how brave and strong I had to be! I had terrible veins for blood taking so I had obviously followed in my grandmother's footsteps and ended up with poor veins. I used all my energy to be strong when the nurse tried constantly to get blood. Thankfully, by the end of the ordeal, the nurse made me a fabulous stick figure type doll that was made with everything to do with blood taking! All except the needle itself, thank goodness. Even to this day, I will never forget that doll. Although I will say that this doll, although I was amazed by it, she certainly was not my favourite or a doll I wanted to cuddle.

After days waiting for the results, Mum and Dad were called by my doctor in Manly and were asked to take me to his surgery for the results of the blood tests. His surgery was a block back from the Manly Ferry Terminal and I remember we always needed to park a few streets away as the commuters would park as close to the ferry terminal as they could for their daily commute from Manly to Circular Quay at Sydney Wharf.

During our appointment, the doctor informed Mum and Dad that their only child was diagnosed with Type 1 diabetes. Although Mum and Dad had a feeling that this was the case, the words coming from the doctor was devastating news for them. Dad had a reasonable amount of knowledge, although limited knowledge, in fact, about diabetes. As both his parents suffered this debilitating disorder, he was knowledgeable enough to know that this disorder would change not only my life but his and Mum's life forever.

Mum was always very good at cooking with a balanced diet and very limited fats in mind. We would always have plenty of vegetables and only on special occasions would we have anything deep fried. The diet side of diabetes was not a major worry for Mum however the concerns about urine testing several times a day and learning how to administer my one needle per day was a major factor and created many months of sleepless nights for both Mum and Dad. It was not just about urine testing and needles, it was also about sterilising needles and syringes, how would I manage at school, hypos, exercise levels, and probably the most important part was the acceptance from people and how they would interpret what their young daughter with diabetes was about.

CHAPTER 8

# WORKSHOP UNDER THE HOUSE

Prior to my fifth birthday, I always remember spending time in my Dad's workshop which he had built under our house. The house was positioned in a cul-de-sac on quite a steep block. It had three bedrooms, a bathroom, an ensuite, lounge room and dining room, together with a double garage. It was red brick with a very steep, curvy driveway. Dad planted two trees in the front garden as a tribute to his parents. Both these trees were a major feature at the front of the house and softened the red bricks with the different coloured green. The larger taller tree was a dark green colour, and this represented my grandfather. The smaller tree which was a softer green was a tribute to my grandmother. On the other side of the driveway, there were plants of many different shapes and sizes that provided some privacy from the next-door neighbours. The front five steps, which were concrete, lead to the front door which had a feature of a large square stainless-steel doorknob. Very typically 1960's. The backyard was extremely steep and had a leafy garden with winding steps that went to the clothesline on the hill. Beyond that was a 40-foot overhanging rock.

My Dad had a great idea of creating his own workshop which he made from the brick piers that held up the floor of the house. There were lots of little hidden alcoves which made a perfect workshop for Dad. He made use of every little nook and cranny that he could find within the confines of the area under the house. Every piece of tooling, every electronic component had its own area. I would spend hours with Dad in his workshop. Dad would show me how to solder. To this day, I can always remember my Dad telling me that a soldering iron could burn me so be very careful, as I watched intently how my Dad could solder. Dad set up a work bench for me which was lower than Dad's benches. He set up a light, a soldering iron, solder, some electronic parts, a printed circuit board and some cutters for the wires and solder. The parts were in a little parts divider and Dad had numbered the dividers and had written on the stickers what each part was. I was only allowed to use the soldering iron under very strict supervision and my Dad was a perfect teacher of my newfound love of electronics.

# CHAPTER 9

# SCHOOL OF ELECTRONICS

This new electronic knowledge, although very basic at such a young age assisted me later in my school years at St Lukes Girls School, on Sydney's beautiful Northern Beaches. It became something that my science teacher took interest in. She asked if I would ask my Dad if he would be interested in spending one afternoon a week in the science room to teach the girls about electronics. I had spoken in class about my Dad teaching me how to solder and how to understand the terminology and colours associated with electronic parts such as diodes and resistors.

Dad jumped at the idea, and I was his second in charge to make sure each student had the correct resistors and could solder properly, carefully, and safely. There were about twelve girls who were interested and as the class was an after-school learning experience, they were all wanting to spend one afternoon per week staying back for an hour and a half to learn all that my Dad could teach them.

This continued for approximately two school terms and the following year my science teacher left and none of the other science teachers were interested to carry it on. Sadly, in those days, it was due to the fact they did not think girls would or should work in electronics.

## CHAPTER 10

# MY FIRST JOB

I remember going to work with my Mum during school holidays. She worked as the Managing Directors personal assistant/secretary at a company called "Suntester" which was located at Ryde. This was a company that manufactured and repaired timing equipment for cars. I was still very young and although people were reasonably understanding of my medical requirements as a Diabetic, it was hard for my Mum to leave me with anyone at all really. Dad and Mum had been in Australia for many years by now and although Mum's brother and sister-in-law had also immigrated to Australia from England, they did not live very close, so they were unable to look after me during the day. Mum spoke with her boss, and he was happy for me to go to work with her during school holidays.

I always remember that he would call me into his office on the Monday morning. I would sit in a chair that was probably about five times the size of me. Mum's boss had a huge swinging, rocking type chair that towered over his head whilst sitting in it. His desk was very large, and it made me feel very nervous. Mum's boss was called "Mr Tancred". I always called him "Mr Tancred" as in the 1960's and 70's, it was good manners and the correct thing to do.

The story of Mr Tancred went back many years as it was Mr Tancred and his wife that looked after me at birth so Mum could maintain her health during her breast cancer threat. I suppose he was more than happy to take me under his wing as a little girl, after all, I was the baby that kept him awake five years earlier.

Mr Tancred would give me a list of jobs he would like me to do. I would take my little "Holly Hobby" notebook and pencil into his office, and he would give me a list of jobs. When I look back now, I clearly remember not knowing what he meant half the time, let alone knowing how to write it or spell it! My list included jobs such as * putting stamps on the envelopes. * finding out what biscuits my Mum's work mates wanted for morning tea. * opening the mail that my Mum received. * making sure there was toilet paper in the toilets!!

My Mum had asked Mr Tancred to give me jobs to help her at work so after about five minutes of writing what I did not even know I was writing, trying to look grown up to Mr Tancred, I would come back out to Mum's desk, and she would go through the list with me.

At the end of each week, Mr Tancred would call me into his office, and he would hand me a very small dark yellow envelope. To my amazement, the envelope had my name on it. It had big capital letters "LISA." The first time he gave me the envelope, I really did not understand what it was. At the age of five or six, your mind does not really understand very much, very clearly, at all. I raced out to Mum's desk and gave her the envelope that Mr Tancred had given to me. Mum knew that he had planned to give me lessons on what working and doing tasks meant and although I did not know it at the time my Mum had set it up. I remember getting a $1 note in my little yellow envelope. To me that was a King's ransom and in the early 1970's, it was a $1 note, not a coin.

To this day, I have Mr Tancred, my Mum, and my working with Dad in his workshop, to thank for my work ethic.

Mum left her job with Mr Tancred after many years of working for him. She was finding that the hour-long travel to work and then another hour's travel home every day was taking its toll on her. She was heartbroken as Mr Tancred and his wife were dear friends and she absolutely loved her job. She was lucky enough to find a job in the office with a company called Bandag Tyres. It was closer to home and fortunately, her new boss was just as fabulous as Mr Tancred. Even to the point where again, I was allowed to go to work with Mum during school holidays and even when I was sick. His three sons worked in the business too and I still to this day remember all three of them allowing me to help them with their work. Mum was there for many years, and it was a job she loved. She also met Alan Grice, the race car driver.

CHAPTER 11

# LIVING WITH DIABETES

As the years went on, my diabetes was something that totally absorbed my every day and night. I would have to sleep, play, and eat in my diabetic world. The stress on Mum and Dad was massive and certainly something that required all of us to adapt to a new lifestyle as well as a new timetable. At the age of nine, I went to a diabetic camp. This was a yearly camp which was designed to teach young children how to look after their diabetes without needing the constant care of parents. It was also a camp in which they would train young and newly diagnosed children how to do their own needles and urine testing. It was set up in a dormitory style so all the girls would sleep in one large room and all the boys would sleep in a separate large room. I seem to remember there were about 20 or 30 of each gender. They would teach you about food groups, carbohydrates and there was always something fabulous to do like bush walking, swimming, exercise activities as well as a great craft room. There was even a large selection of games to play.

School was a challenge for a child with diabetes. I specifically remember one horrible time in primary school where a boy punched me in my upper arm because he knew I had to put needles in my arm. He was duly punished with a few strikes of the cane so gladly neither him, nor any other boy ever tried to hurt me again.

I remember having to have morning tea and lunch at school during different times to the normal school recess and lunch. I would need to go out of the classroom at 10am and 12.30. This meant I would be excused from the classroom, sadly interrupting the entire class, when the teacher would say "Lisa, time for your morning tea or lunch." I would then come back into the classroom and very shortly after my return, the class would be sent out for our break.

This was extremely bad in my first years in high school as the other kids, not knowing how hard it was living with diabetes, would cruelly pick on and bully me for needing to leave the classroom early. I even got picked on for needing to go to the staff room for sugar, due to a hypo. Thankfully, I was aware of how I felt when a hypo came on so the teachers would allow me to go to the staff room. I was the only student that was allowed into the teachers' staff room and the staff would sit me down and make me a drink of warm water with sugar. The torment from the other students became increasingly punishing for me. Kids would even superglue my locker shut so I could not access my morning tea, lunch and even jellybeans if I needed them in case of a hypo.

Sadly, kids can be very cruel. This continued for several years and ironically, some of those "kids" became great friends in my early twenties.

I also remember a very unexpected occurrence during a sleepover at my next-door neighbour's house. Her name was Maria, and she was the best neighbour I could ask for in my young years. Maria also suffered a life changing condition as she was born deaf. We were lucky enough to spend most of our weekends playing together and learning to understand each other's disorders. I quickly learnt to speak clearly with my lips so she could understand me, and with her enhanced intuition, she knew me well enough to know when I needed food and even if I was going into a mild hypo. I taught her what hypo meant and I would right down words and she taught me how to move my mouth so she could clearly understand lip movements. A perfect lesson in lipreading/speaking so it was quite a match made in heaven for two young friends.

I had a little dog called Sloopy. He was my very first dog and was also my best friend. He was a beagle cross kelpie, but we called him a Heinz 57 variety dog as he seemed to have a bit of everything in his breed. He was a beautiful dog although he did have a slight devilish but adorably cute personality. He once followed me to school and in assembly, he jumped on the headmaster's knee. All the kids were in hysterics with laughter however the headmaster did not see the funny side and expelled poor Sloopy from school. Sloopy was extremely intuitive with alerting Mum and Dad when I was having a hypo overnight. He would sleep next to my bed and would only leave me if he sensed I was having a hypo. Sloopy would race into Mum and Dad's bedroom and wake them up to alert them to my hypo. Every single time, his intuition was correct. This was also something that, thankfully, was able to put Mum and Dad's mind at rest overnight. Fast forward to today, I now own a beautiful dog called Pilot and luckily, she has also taken on the same intuitive nature as Sloopy by alerting my family when I am affected by a hypo.

Maria and I would often set up a little circus in her front yard. We would find anything we could either in her Dad's garage or my Dad's garage and set up a few different mazes for Sloopy to wander through. We would use treats to get him to do whatever trick he needed to do. It worked wonders and we spent many hours a weekend doing the same thing. We were both worried that Sloopy would get dizzy doing the same path through the maze, so we decided to get him to do the maze the other way around.

As we lived in a cul-de-sac and without the worry of traffic we would ride our bikes, roller skates and scooters every day and spent many fun filled hours together.

Both our Mums realised that sleepovers were a very important part of growing up. Maria's Mum said she was happy for me to stay overnight. I do honestly think that she realised that Mum and Dad never got much sleep worrying about me going into a hypo or hyper and although they were both constantly giving the correct insulin dose and food intake, a diabetics body would often do its own thing!

"No problem", my friend's Mum said to my Mum. "Lisa is more than welcome to stay. You and Stan have a night off and if I need you, I will ring or knock on the door". Maria's Mum was a breath of fresh air for my Mum as Mum rarely had a break from looking after me with diabetes. As Maria was deaf, it was pointless expecting her to hear me if I was having a bad hypo. Her Mum promised Mum she would keep her ears and eyes open for my very first sleepover without Mum and Dad. Maria and I were both very excited.

Sadly, in the very early hours of the morning the inevitable happened and Mum and Dad were woken by a phone call from Maria's Mum saying that I wasn't good. I had obviously had the most exciting sleep over and with all the physical and mental energy used earlier that night, my body had used too much sugar and I went into a bad hypo. Unfortunately, it was the last sleep over I had for many years after.

CHAPTER 12

# PARTY TIME

In my early years of becoming a diabetic, life was tough. My Mum would have to weigh all the food she gave me to make sure the amount of carbohydrate was correct. I remember Mum feeling sorry for me that I could not eat chocolate, so she bought all the necessary ingredients and made me diabetic chocolate. It was simply sugar free chocolate and I was so excited for my afternoon teatime, which was always 3.30pm on the dot.

My Mum was just as excited as I was. Not only to taste the chocolate but also to see that I could experience the same things other kids of my age were experiencing and what they were able to have when I was sadly unable to have such treats being a diabetic.

I always remember Dad would buy me a "flake" chocolate bar as a special treat and sadly when I became a diabetic, this treat ended. Unfortunately, when I was able to try the chocolate that Mum had spent so much time making, it was horrible. Artificial sweeteners were not like they are today, so the taste was bitter and horrible enough to throw it straight into the garbage bin. Mum was heartbroken as her little girl was unable to experience chocolate like she was used to. Mum also attempted to make me cakes with artificial sweetener however, sadly, they were not very nice at all.

Birthday parties were always very difficult, not only for me but for Mum. She would take me to the party and confirm with my friends' Mum that I should not have any sweet party food." This broke her heart, but it was the only way I could attend the party and keep my levels of carbohydrate and sugar within the proper boundaries.

I was only allowed to have vegemite or peanut butter sandwiches. It was quite sad for a young child watching all her friends go crazy on all the sweet party food. It got to the point where my friend's parents thought it was best that I did not go to the parties as fairy bread and chocolate crackles did not fit with the diet requirements I should have. It was also a major responsibility for the mother of my friend having the birthday. She would be more concerned about what I was going to eat, rather than the party itself. They also felt extremely sorry for me that as a young child, I was missing out on party food.

Mum was absolutely devastated with this and after a few years, she finally said that I could eat a very small amount of the party food and she would deal with the repercussions after the party. This would have meant high sugar implications as party food for young children in the 1970's, always included fairy bread, chocolate crackles, freckles, and lolly snakes.

Another extraordinarily strong memory of being a young and newly diagnosed diabetic was a party at the Camperdown Children's Hospital, otherwise known as The Royal Alexandra Hospital for Children. The hospital was in Sydney, so it was an hour and a half drive from our home. I do not remember if the party was for any specific occasion however, I do remember there was a hat parade. Mum thought of the brilliant idea of creating a diabetic scene on my hat. My Mum not only made the best birthday cakes, but she also had quite a creative and extremely thoughtful imagination. Her idea was a set of weight scales with needles, insulin and urine testing tablets, strips, test tubes on one side of the scales and a slice of bread, a piece of fruit and some jellybeans on the other side. We were able to find some plastic scales in a toy shop so thankfully they were not heavy. Mum and I worked hard and meticulously by creating an absolute masterpiece of a hat. My Mum's brilliant idea awarded me first place. Overly exciting for a young girl whose everyday life was about having to endure urine tests, needles, and very controlled food intake.

CHAPTER 13

# EARLY MANAGEMENT

The only way to check the amount of sugar in your body in the early 1970's was urine testing. This was the only option when living at home and out of the hospital environment. I always remember having to put five drops of urine in a test tube that had been boiled for sanitising and then placing a tablet into the urine and shaking it. After a brief time, the contents of the test tube would change colour. Whatever colour was in the test tube would be checked against a colour graph on the outside of the urine test bottle. This would then indicate how much sugar was in your body.

Unfortunately, urine testing was not a perfectly accurate way of checking sugar levels. Urine testing was sometimes messy as accidental spillage could sometimes occur and although it gave a vague indication of whether the sugar level was low or high, it was not an exact science. Also, often urine is held in your bladder for a considerable amount of time which could mean that your actual sugar level may be quite different from the time you did the urine test. The only way to accurately monitor glucose levels was blood testing and at this time could only be done by a doctor or qualified professional at the hospital or a laboratory.

Mum and Dad would also have to boil my glass syringes and stainless steel re-usable needles for insulin injection. Thankfully, my Godfather, good old Uncle Barry was a sheet metal worker so he made a stainless-steel container that had a slide out lid that Mum and Dad could put my glass syringes and re-usable needles in for boiling and sanitising to prevent any infections to the injection site. As the needles were re-usable, they were often blunt and would hurt increasingly as they became old and used.

My Dad had worked on reflectance meters in his early working years and was fluent with his knowledge and the association with being able to use a reflectance meter to monitor blood sugar levels. This is what they did with the hospital machine's so Dad spent many hours using his reflectance meter and electronics knowledge so therefore was fully aware of how the hospital machines worked. He totally understood the technology and knew exactly how it worked.

CHAPTER 14

# PHENOMENON IN THE MAKING

One specific week in 1978, my Dad spent more than the usual amount of time he would normally spend in his workshop underneath the house. At night, Mum would feed us dinner, which was always a sit-down meal at the table. It was Dad's routine to go from dinner to his workshop to either repair, create or make something from all his electronic parts. My Dad would always whistle when he was creating something. It was only when he was creating, the repairs did not quite give him the enthusiasm that creating electronic gadgets gave him. He did not whistle any specific song, but he was always in key and always made everything he whistled sound like an incredible orchestra. During this one week, Dad would spend more time in his workshop. His whistling became stronger, and more tune varied, and he went quiet at the dinner table. Mum and I were not really thinking anything other than maybe he was simply enjoying his dinners increasingly, even though Mum wasn't really cooking anything unusual or different. My Dad never had a bad mood. He was always happy, whistling and simply loved his life. He was always very level-headed and very approachable about absolutely anything. Both Mum and I wondered, but were not worried, about what was keeping him so quiet and focused.

Dad would always draw diagrams of electronic circuit boards and being an electronics engineer, to both Mum and I, as well as anyone else that viewed them, they were simply a diagram of squiggly lines, straight lines, and numbers. If I ever asked Dad what a particular diagram was, he would produce the most amazing, straight forward, explanatory definition. He would explain how it worked and what components he would use and why he would use them.

The diagrams were becoming more detailed, and the quantity of diagrams went from only a few in that week to a small exercise book full of Dad's electronic circuit board diagrams. We also noticed Dad had a look of determination on his face so we both knew that all of Dad's concentration was going into something important. This made Mum and I realise that whatever Dad was creating, it had to be something truly remarkable. We both also knew that to pressure Dad for information about this project was useless as Dad would always let you know about what he was thinking or creating when he had it perfectly clear in his own mind.

Whatever Dad was working on was consuming him. Dad came up to the house particularly late for dinner one night and Mum had even gone to the workshop to see if he was OK. He told her he was almost ready to come upstairs for dinner so give him some time and he would be up soon. In those days, reheating food was not an easy task so Mum was concerned her cooking would end up a ruined plate of freshly cooked food as it sat in the oven with aluminium foil over it for quite some time. We always ate dinner about 5.30 in the afternoon as in the 1970's, with the limited technology available for diabetes management, time was a major component of insulin control and food. It was always to the minute that food would be eaten and the amount of food, mainly carbohydrate, was extremely tightly controlled.

At the age of twelve, I would usually go to bed about 8.30pm. This one night, Dad came upstairs from his workshop about 8pm. He was not interested in dinner but did have a tray of electronic components as well as other parts that I had never seen before. I always tested my sugar level before bed using the hospital machine that we got from my Endocrinologist Martin Silink. Martin had loaned a hospital machine to Mum and Dad as he was aware that they were struggling to manage my glucose levels using urine testing. Martin realised that blood glucose testing, which was being carried out in the hospital, was an instant result and this was having great success with the management of his patients that had difficulty controlling their diabetes.

Dad put the tray on the dining table and asked me to give him the strip with which I put the finger prick of blood onto. This is what I had to do to get the result of my sugar level using the hospital machine. Mum and I questioned why he wanted the strip, and the next thing we looked on as Dad placed the blood glucose strip into some contraption sitting on the tray that Dad had brought up from his workshop. Dad then pressed a button and a meter that he had wired up gave some form of reading. When Mum and I asked what he was doing, he then took the strip out of his contraption and placed it in the hospital machine. He then said, "IT WORKS!".

My Dad had spent only one week in his workshop and during this one momentous week, he had through his immense knowledge and background in electronics created the world's first home blood glucose monitor.

He certainly did not realise what he had created as he only did it to keep me out of hospital and have something at home that could read the direct amount of sugar in the blood. Something that urine testing did not offer safely or accurately. Dad's mind never stopped and often during this time, he would come upstairs in the early hours of the morning to finally get some sleep before another full day at work.

CHAPTER 15

# LET'S MANUFACTURE THIS CREATION

My Dad still worked at Hanimex, Brookvale at this time. Thankfully, it wasn't far from where we lived so he did have the benefit of being able to leave home a little later. Dad's brain was always developing something new and worthwhile. He had a natural ability to also be able to repair absolutely anything that did not work.

Once Dad had worked out the electronics of the glucose tester, he then moved on to make a machine that would vacuum form the cases to hold the electronics and batteries in place. My memory of this was a pump and some tubing, together with a beer keg. My Dad did not drink alcohol, so I am amazed how he even produced the idea of a beer keg. Dad also had to make a bracket to hold the PVC plastic sheets in place so he could place the hot PVC over the mould and then press the foot pedal which sucked the hot PVC over the mould. Dad also made the mould for the vacuum former. He had a metal lathe in his workshop, so he designed the complete casing mould and made it himself with his lathe. A brilliant and diverse man...

Dad made the very first machine and still to this day is my pride and joy. Dad had written in black indelible texter "LISA's – SAVE". It was the prototype and although the test strips for the prototype are no longer available, it would still be working and accurate today, even after 40 odd years. I will not let this machine out of my sight, and I keep it in my Mums little safe. Dad made everything for this machine by hand. He did get stickers made to place inside the battery compartment so you could see which way to insert the batteries as well as getting the meters printed to show where the sugar level sat. Low, medium, and high range were determined by bold lines on the meter.

He had thought of absolutely everything to make the machine easy to use, easy to see and something you could take anywhere with you. Dad had always wanted to go camping and had built a campervan to go on the top of his Toyota Ute. That is when seats in a Ute were for three people, which enabled our family of three to go in the campervan for adventures. He made the campervan from sheet metal, and he welded, and pop riveted the entire van from scratch. It had a queen-sized bed over the Ute cabin, it had a small stainless-steel sink, a small fridge with a freezer, two single beds which were set up as bunks and plenty of storage. Therefore, this led Dad to decide the glucose testers should be not only be mains power operated but also battery operated.

Although the first machine was about the size of a brick, it was lightweight and had a lid which was made of clear, thick plastic. This protected the meter, the calibration knobs, and the test strip slide insert. The test strip slide insert is the part where the test strip was placed into the machine for reading glucose levels. He had even made the machine with a battery safety layer which would prevent any battery corrosion damaging the internal electronics and in turn, the accuracy of the machine.

We spent many days making the trip to the Royal Alexandra Hospital for Children. Over the years, I spent many horrible weeks as an admitted patient and was extremely closely monitored to get my sugar levels and insulin dosages perfectly aligned. The testing in the hospital was always via a canular into the vein in my arm which would stay there for a week or more. I remember spending time, over the duration of each admission, in a different ward. The one I particularly remember was a hospital ward down the very back of the hospital. It had a large and exceptionally long concrete balcony which overlooked amazingly green trees which always had birds singing in them. This was known as "Sailing League Ward". I do not know where the name came from however, I always remember it as the vein blood room. Certainly not a wonderful place to be however all the kids in this ward were there for close monitoring of blood testing. I remember the bath in this ward was extremely large and very deep. As I was there during the age of 7 to 11, the bath was the only thing that I was happy to be there for. It was like a swimming pool and was built up in the middle of the bathroom. I did meet several kids in Sailing League Ward, and we all made the most of the time we were there. They had games, books, colouring in, posters on the wall and a TV which was large enough for us all to sit around and watch.

The Royal Alexandra Hospital for Children sat very proudly on a magnificent block of land. It was a large hospital, the main part of the building was built of sandstone and was, over the years, increased in size by several different structures, these new buildings were a combination of additions to the original section as well as separate individual buildings around the grounds which were built from brick and timber. Some parts were connected by a closed in and covered walkway. Perfect for when the weather was horrible, and the rain was torrential.

This one morning we made the trip to the Royal Alexandra Hospital for Children. The trip to the hospital was to not only have my usual check-up but this was the time Dad was going to show my doctor his creation of a blood glucose tester. It was quite exciting when Dad explained to my doctor how the blood glucose machine worked. Dad certainly knew his stuff! My doctor was Martin Silink. Martin was the Head of Endocrinology at the children's hospital in Sydney and after viewing and learning about what Dad had created, he was speechless and quite overwhelmed at what he was seeing. Obviously, it was important that the machine was tested for accuracy, and this is something Martin took upon himself by making sure the machine was extremely accurate. Clearly, if he were to use the machines on his patients, he needed a guarantee of its accuracy.

The tests for accuracy were initially carried out at the Royal Alexandra Hospital for Children in "Sailing League Ward" which was known as the metabolic ward of the hospital. Dad's machines were tested, and with these results was irreputable proof that the machine that Dad had created was 99 + % accurate. Martin Silink had conducted the tests and produced a report on the accuracy of Dad's invention. Within minutes of it being approved by the hospital management, Martin ordered thirty machines for use in the clinic on the children with difficult to control diabetes. These were the patients that often struggled to maintain a stable sugar level. Martin had arranged approval for the hospital to provide the funds for Dad to produce these machines and by the end of 1979, Martin Silink had ordered a machine for every child in the clinic needing one. He also ordered machines for the wards and emergency department.

Martin could see the amazing benefits that regular home blood glucose monitoring would have in helping his young patients. It was incredible that Martin Silink received some controversial censure as it was thought, by some, that enforcing children to prick their finger every day was cruel. Sadly, the people that felt this way had not given any consideration to the fact that home blood glucose monitoring was an immediate and accurate measure of sugar levels, so much better than urine testing which was the current standard form of monitoring glucose. Certainly, this new form of monitoring would be more than beneficial to not only immediate control but also long-term outcomes. Also, any person, whether a child or an adult, would not flinch at a finger prick when they were so used to insulin injections.

Martin was also assisted with his work by Margaret McGill. Margaret was the Diabetes Educator at the Royal Alexandra Hospital for Children and was in fact the very first Paediatric Diabetes Educator in Australia. They were a formidable team and together they committed their efforts to ensuring that every diabetic child they cared for had complete management of their diabetes and, were the proud owners of one of Dad's home blood glucose testers. Many years later Martin was honoured with the title of "Professor" and Margaret with the title of "Associate Professor". They worked tirelessly, not only as a team but also individually and their hard work was certainly rewarded with such a deserving and prestigious title. It was obvious that they loved their work with children with diabetes and their families.

Over the following months, the news throughout the Sydney hospital system was that an affordable home glucose tester had just been invented. Mum and Dad were inundated with calls from newspapers, magazines and television stations wanting all the information available on the testers. The tester orders were coming through thick and fast from individual people willing to do anything to get their hands on one of my Dad's machines. It was at this point of time that Dad realised that he was unable to continue working at Hanimex and needed to leave his job and concentrate 100% on manufacturing his invention.

The orders for glucose testers intensified and my poor Mum was forced to cook either stove top dinners, microwave food or buy take away. Her oven was used 14 hours a day to heat the Perspex to make the cases for the testers. This continued for months, and Dad overworked my Mum's oven so much that it blew up and it set on fire. Dad's workshop also became too small to produce the hundreds and hundreds of testers as the equipment was now being ordered by the thousands. We had diodes, capacitors, circuit boards, cases, transformers, and packaging products which took up every single square inch of Dad's workshop.

Mum and Dad realised that they needed a factory as the orders were now coming from interstate, England, Russia, America, in fact all over the world. Dad was overwhelmed with the orders and was in a situation where he was left with no other option than to rent a factory in Dee Why on the Northern Beaches of Sydney.

The factory was situated behind a fish shop so the smell was not great but every so often Mum would get their seafood for dinner. Great food, great owners of the fish shop and some memories of a time in our lives that will never be forgotten.

Dad knew that he needed a business name and knew that the business needed to be a company. Several names came into question until Dad, as he always had his whistling whilst thinking mannerism; got his usual pitch about his whistling and came up with the idea of naming his new business "Australian BIO Transducers". He registered the name Ligg Pty Ltd trading as Australian BIO Transducers. This was registered in 1979. I often wondered where the name Australian BIO Transducers came from and what it meant. Dad explained that although he was English, it was important that the word Australian was in the name as both Mum and Dad were proud naturalised Australian residents. Also, the world's first home glucose tester was an invention created in Australia. BIO means life so he felt this was a machine that would provide a strong and long life for any diabetic who would now be able to monitor their own blood glucose levels at home. Transducer is a device that is used to detect a signal or energy and convert it from its original form to the desired form or otherwise a device that converts variations in a physical quantity. Therefore, to Dad, this meant that the electronics that he used in his glucose testers would simply convert to a blood glucose result. I still, to this day, think Dad's business name is something that was extremely well thought of and decided upon, and the name became an extremely well-known entity in the diabetes world.

Mum and Dad worked tirelessly to run the business and incredibly tried to keep everyone who ordered a machine on a short waiting time for delivery of their purchase. Mum spent many hours dealing with the post office as well as courier companies, with the aim to have delivery of the glucose testers the quickest, cheapest, and most efficient delivery possible.

Diabetes Australia, which was then known as the Diabetic Association, had an office in Pitt Street Sydney. A small organisation at the time, however, this was an organisation that had been running for a few decades at this stage, so it was paramount that we worked very closely with them as they were an extremely important part in the lives of diabetics. It was also due to our relationship with Diabetes Australia that later in time I was proud to be appointed a Diabetes Australia Ambassador. The building which housed their office in Sydney was extremely old and staged a beautifully presented stone façade. The lift used to access the office from the ground floor, was old and quite scary to use. I will say though, never once in the time either Mum, Dad or I used it, did it break down. I am very thankful for that as I am extremely claustrophobic and the thought of being stuck in a lift is something I certainly would not be able to deal with.

As the orders were continually coming through for the glucose testers, it was so busy that it got to the point where Dad had to make the decision that only pregnant woman and children could get a tester quickly. Otherwise, the wait was approximately 3 weeks. With orders and supply going crazy, Dad was contacted by a woman that begged him to supply her daughter with a glucose tester. She cried on the phone and said that her diabetic daughter had lost several pregnancies due to diabetes. My Dad had a heart of gold and with this phone call, he made an extra attempt to make sure the young woman was in supply of a machine within a couple of days.

Approximately 12 months later, Mum and Dad had a lady come into the factory with a pram and her Mum. It was the woman that Dad got the call about. They were so grateful for the glucose tester, and she wanted Dad to know that without his invention and his willingness to help wherever he could to supply her with a machine so promptly, she would not be pushing a pram.

This news of a successful pregnancy brought tears to my Dad's eyes. My Dad was the humblest human being I knew and never once did he think of himself as being a hero. I really do not think he ever truly realised what a phenomenon he had created. To this day, I remember him saying he only did it for me.

After many sleepless nights and extremely long hours and weeks, Mum and Dad were taking the phenomenal interest in his invention one day at a time. I was 12 years old at this stage and although I could help with packing of the testers and doing the postage side of the business, there was not much else I could do. I was at school so had homework and although Dad had taught me to solder, I could not help with any more than what I was doing. I used to catch the bus home from school, and it was then just a small walk from the bus stop to home. I would go home, do my homework, and then cook Mum and Dad dinner for when they got home about 7pm. It was at this point that I understood what a Mum did. Cooking, washing, folding, cleaning, shopping together with a full-time job of running a business that created a mammoth task for both Mum and Dad. I tried to take as much load from Mum with the house but at such a youthful age, whatever I attempted probably wasn't the best effort. Mum was always incredibly grateful as she barely had the time to scratch.

Within a few months of starting the glucose testers, my Dad's niece, my cousin Linda, asked if I could be her bridesmaid. She lived in England and although the timing was not particularly good for Mum to leave, Dad felt it was important for me to be my cousin's bridesmaid. My Dad's sister, Ada, Linda's mother, had flown over from England when I was first diagnosed as she understood what turmoil Mum and Dad would be going through after diabetes claimed the lives of my Dad and Aunty Ada's parents. Mum flew with me over to England for Linda's wedding and both Mum and Dad decided to take me out of school for several months, not only to attend the wedding but to also visit my extended British family. Mum had not seen her sister for many years, and it was also an opportunity to visit some of my cousins that I had never met. With schoolwork carefully packed in my suitcase, Mum and I made the nearly 24-hour long-haul flight to Heathrow Airport in England, and we were very warmly welcomed by my Aunty Ada on our arrival.

During the time we spent in England, Mum decided to take the glucose tester to some of the hospitals in England. They also were totally amazed at what my Dad had created and after the hospitals did their own homework on accuracy etc, they all ordered glucose testers for not only the hospitals but also for their patients.

For many years, our little family business was something that had been created out of my Dad's brilliant mind. We were continuously looking at how we could increase the awareness of the importance of home blood glucose testing. Dad was constantly approached by the media, and it was suggested that Dad be a contestant on the channel 9 program showcasing new Australian inventions called "What'll they think of next". Dad became a contestant on the show and was awarded a first-place tie. One of the shows judges were so impressed with Dad's invention that they decided to assist by volunteering and offered to attend blood screening in several locations around Sydney. The screening stations were set up with the help of Diabetes Australia as they felt awareness was important and for people to be able to have their blood glucose levels checked extremely quickly and effortlessly.

It was alarmingly surprising how many people presented with high glucose levels and did not even know it. The public awareness became surreal and once again, my Dad's invention would continue to help the general public be able to get their glucose levels checked at various set ups around not only Sydney but also country towns across Australia. The blood screening continued for months and this, together with Dad's glucose tester, immediately dropped the number of admissions to hospitals around the globe from long term diabetic complications.

Glucose levels were monitored amazingly fast and in an extremely accurate and very cheap manner. The awareness became an overnight success, and I will always say that my Dad's invention was the greatest thing since insulin in a diabetic's life. It enabled a diabetic to manage their own glucose levels daily and report these results back to their doctor. The doctor knew these results were accurate and instant, no matter what time of day or night. This allowed a diabetic to take more control of their glucose levels and with the help of their doctor and education, a diabetic could take major stress off the hospital system and government spending.

To give an idea of the stress that glucose testing took from the medical system, in 1978/79 the thirty children that were initially given the first thirty glucose testers had collectively spent 360 days in hospital. In the following year, the same thirty children using the glucose testers only spent 55 days collectively in hospital. This result was based on only thirty children so the number of diabetics around the world and the number of days that home glucose testing was being carried out was reducing hospital admissions dramatically.

The business continued for many years supplying glucose testers to diabetics in every corner of the globe. Over the years, Dad had created new and improved models to keep up with technology and, also wanted to make the testers smaller and lighter. He spent any profits he made from the sales of previous models of testers and would use this to produce new testers.

CHAPTER 16

# NEW AND IMPROVED MODELS

The initial testers were powered by a transformer which would plug into a standard power point, together with the ability to be run from either a cigarette lighter or simple C sized batteries. This was revolutionary as prior to Dad's invention, the hospital machines were only mains powered. This meant that you could be in the middle of the bush or on a boat and still be able to check your own blood glucose levels. As time progressed, Dad decided to make the glucose testers so they could be powered not by large and heavy C sized batteries but also by AA batteries. This was a remarkable achievement as this also meant that the glucose testers could be made smaller and without the extra weight of adding the larger, heavier C sized batteries.

Dad's next brilliant but necessary idea was to make the glucose testers so they could be operated using re-chargeable batteries. This was important to Dad as he always realised that the cost of living with diabetes was extremely high, not only for the insulin but also for the needles, the test strips as well as the cost of necessary doctors' appointments so Dad wanted people to not have the additional cost of disposable batteries. A small consideration to some but my Dad was always thinking about people not being able to get batteries when they required them. He would always be thinking ahead which is what made his many glucose tester models so remarkable in its time.

Dad had thought about every person with his glucose tester manufacture. He had a girl contact him saying that she could not read the meter on the machine, therefore, not being able to know exactly what her glucose level was. My Dad, being the brilliant man that he was, used his electronic knowledge and within a week, had created a glucose tester which used coloured lights to show what a person's glucose level was. This was not suitable for blind people however poor vision was often a sign of poor diabetic sugar level control and people with bad vision could still see colour. Dad therefore made the brilliant decision that green would represent a low to good zone, amber would represent the mid glucose levels and red would represent the high to highest level. Depending on what side of the machine the green, amber, or red showed up would determine where the sugar level was.

This was tried and tested and the new coloured light model of glucose tester, that Dad had caringly dedicated his thoughts and knowledge to, was a game changer for diabetics with poor eyesight. He then set out to make a glucose tester give out a signal which was used for blind diabetics. Another brilliant idea. He then went on to invent a device which would enable a blind person to be able to prick their finger and place the drop of blood onto the pad of the test strip. This was an impossible task for a person with poor eyesight or no eyesight at all.

Not only did Dad's glucose testers reduce the amount of admissions to hospitals around the world due to diabetic illness and complications, also the amount of people with diabetic eye damage were gradually reducing in numbers. People that had previously suffered poor vision from high sugar levels were able to, in some cases, repair their eye damage by maintaining excellent control of their sugars.

CHAPTER 17

# OTHER INTERESTS

Dad was a HAM radio operator. It was a hobby he had enjoyed for years. We lived on the top of a hill in Wheeler Heights. Not only did Dad have his under the house workshop but he had purposely built a garden shed on the top of the rock in the back yard. This little garden shed was his radio shed. Dad had made his HAM radio aerial out of random pieces of electronics he had collected for years. He put a motor in it so it would rotate to a certain position to enable him to get better reception for his radio, and the communication it gave him would allow him to speak with people from countries all over the world.

My Dad had built me a cage under the rock that his radio shed was on. My Godfather had bought me a duck called Donald. Dad put wire from the rock to the ground which created a cage that I could stand in. Dad also made a little pool for Donald. It was built out of concrete, and it was big enough for Donald to have a little paddle during the hot months. Donald Duck was my best mate as he would waddle around the back yard following me everywhere I went. We were aware that Donald could be lonely as with Mum and Dad at work and me at school, Donald was home alone during the weekdays, so we decided to get Donald a girlfriend. We called her Daisy. Donald and Daisy did not have any babies, so we often wondered if Daisy was a male. They both lived in their 5-star palatial home for years and then sadly one morning, Dad discovered that Donald had drowned in his pond overnight. We really do not know what had happened to him, but he was in his pond dead. Daisy was fine and healthy and lived for a year after that sad day. I was heartbroken and as there was no evidence of anything breaking through the wire enclosure, we assumed that poor Donald drowned. I can honestly say that I am not sure of anyone saying that a duck drowned. It does sound quite comical however it totally devastated me at the time, and Mum suffered trying to get my sugar levels under any control for weeks due to the emotional turmoil I was suffering.

I will always remember Dad's radio number. It was VK2AYI. I always think of this when I hear the word radio. The AYI at the end of Dads call sign stood for Alpha Yancy India. I would listen to Dad on his radio for hours and at such an early age, I was absolutely amazed how easy it was for Dad to speak to someone on the other side of the world. My Dad also obtained a sound licence in his younger years and although I do not remember any part of his details about this, I do know that his call sign was G3KFM.

My Dad, the brilliant man that he was, was also an automotive mechanical engineer. He loved understanding the knowledge of how a car worked and used this knowledge to rebuild the engine and gear box of a Morris mini. My Godfather Barry, the sheet metal worker, who was also the person my Mum called when she found her stolen car, also had knowledge of engines and gear boxes and together they repaired a mechanically broken little car. Mum's little white mini became her pride and joy, and she even found a long, clear sticker with union jacks on it which Dad placed on the very top of the windscreen. It looked very British! We both went many places in this cute and trustworthy car, a car which never once broke down. Once again, my Dad had repaired and created, using his fabulous knowledge, something that was totally reliable.

CHAPTER 18

# A GROWING BUSINESS

As the business grew and became a worldwide success, sadly, Dad did not get the time or the energy to ever enjoy his radio again. Every spare minute that Dad had was taken up with the business. The orders for Dad's glucose testers were rapidly increasing and it was only a brief period of time before the orders were coming from England, America, Russia, even Lebanon just to name a few.

Most of the Diabetic Association branches were asking for Dad's machines, as well as asking Dad to go and speak at their members nights. This became a monthly occurrence as Dad, Mum and I would pack up for an overnight stay and head to a town many hours away from home. We needed to stay overnight as the meetings were always at night. This enabled the association members to attend as they all had day jobs. I do think, looking back now, that it was really our only way of having a slight break from the intense manufacturing that was absorbing all our time. Mum had spoken with my school about the meetings and explained the situation, thankfully, the teachers were willing to allow me to have a couple of days off once a month on the proviso that I took my homework with me and brought it back fully completed.

Dad's little factory at the back of the fish shop was in a perfect location to walk to absolutely every necessary place our family business needed. There was also a chicken shop on the walkway between the factory and the fish shop. We did not only get the smell of fish, but we would then be welcomed by the most amazing chicken smells as we continued to walk from the fish shop to the main road of Dee Why. They would cook BBQ chickens, hot chips, chicken croquettes, chicken rolls with gravy, tubs of chicken breast pieces in sauces such as mornay, curry, BBQ, satay. In summer, the mixed smells of both the fish shop and chicken shop was not pleasant however in winter, it was a difficult decision for Mum, Dad, and I to decide what to have for dinner on our takeaway nights. The factory was a quick minute's walk from the bus stop, which was the bus route from Wynyard in Sydney via Manly and was the main bus line of the North Shore. This meant that anyone wanting to use public transport could travel to the factory and collect their glucose tester with little effort or trouble.

The factory was a single level brick building. It was long and skinny and had two parking spaces, the front window was covered with a white metal security frame. The building was not massive however it contained all the necessary space for the purpose of building the glucose testers. It had a large assembly room which had a concrete floor and a large window. Although the window was a substantial size and let in good light, Dad needed to install large fluorescent lighting to give maximum coverage to fully bathe the production benches with necessary lighting. He set up shelving at the back of each bench, so the electronic parts and all the necessary items required to build the glucose testers was nearby. Little plastic containers were attached to the shelving on the walls which made assembling the testers a straightforward production line process. Every single item was clearly labelled to help the assembly process of the glucose testers go without a hitch. Each bench had all the necessary tools to build each and every part required for the glucose testers to be manufactured efficiently.

As time went on, Dad rearranged the production room several times. This was due to the fact he would produce a new model of machine and that would mean each model would have a slightly unique way of being assembled. It also meant that different parts would be required for every new model of glucose tester.

The factory had a little kitchenette, which Dad made sure it was fitted out with a microwave, a toaster, and a kettle. It also had a great pantry so there was plenty of room for crockery, cutlery as well as plastic containers for the microwave and storage of food. It did have a decent size fridge which meant the staff that Dad employed could store and cook their lunch and it also allowed Mum to do her grocery shopping when she needed to and keep the cold items in the fridge and freezer until home time. The factory only had one toilet, so everyone had to use the same toilet. It was in a room at the very back of the factory and it was large enough to have a decent sized hand basin.

The storage room at the back of the factory was large enough to keep lots of necessary stock to enable Dad to make thousands of glucose testers and there was even enough room in the storeroom to keep all the packaging items required to box the testers ready for the courier or post office. Once again, every single item was neatly and safely stored, ready for production. Just in front of the storeroom was an office which was big enough for about three desks. It was 1979 so computers had just become something that everyone knew about however few people had one. Mum had to type several documents in the running of the business, so Dad decided to purchase a computer for her to be able to create and print whatever she needed. Mum had not had any computer training as computers were only new and there was little knowledge on how to work them, other than the operator manual which was quite daunting for a first-time user. My Mum was quite a bright spark so after a few attempts, together with a few mistakes, Mum had worked out how to carry out the tasks she needed to type a letter, print it, and save it.

Just next to the office area was a room in which the completed glucose testers were stored and packed. Every single glucose tester had a serial number, and this serial number was not only written on the inside of each tester but also on a little sticker on the base of the machine. The serial number was also stored in a book which was a hardcover foolscap size. An era when A4 size paper was not a major part in an office environment. A4 was then becoming the new standard and to this day foolscap can only be obtained by only a limited specialist paper manufacturer. Mum stored all the information in the foolscap hardcover book. It contained the serial number of the machine, the person who purchased it, the date it was purchased, the date it was checked prior to leaving the factory, also the date and how it was delivered. Mum and Dad named this book the RAHC bible. The "RAHC" stands for Royal Alexandra Hospital for Children, and it was a book which Mum would put in the small safe they had in the storeroom of the factory at the end of every day. It was simply a ledger that contained absolutely every aspect about every single glucose tester that Dad had manufactured, and it was extremely important.

The second desk in the office was set up specifically for our courier to collect the parcels. Mum had another foolscap hard cover book, which was purely for the details of the parcels collected by the courier, including serial number, name, and address of the person the glucose tester was to be delivered to. This also included the collection date. This book was also important to the running of the factory and the business as if anyone mentioned that their glucose tester had not arrived on the arranged delivery time, Mum could check the details and could then follow up with the courier company for clarification of a delivery date. Every single detail of the business was recorded, every item that was in the factory was documented. Mum and Dad did not leave any stone unturned.

CHAPTER 19

# A PERFECT TEAM

Dad was blessed with a great team of workers. Every single one of them gave their all with helping keep the business running without a hitch. They gave their time, their thoughts and suggestions, their laughs and love and the communication between the entire team is something that helped Dad have a very stable and perfectly run business. Dad was a great boss, he would treat all his staff with the utmost respect and along with his kind nature, they would bend over backwards for him. They were all like our family and everyday Mum and Dad were grateful to them for their efforts. Without them, I can honestly say that we could not have managed this business growth ourselves.

I still, to this day, remember Dad's main employees which he had for many years. Mary was involved in the production of every single tester, she was a fantastic person for the job as she was methodical and very patient, which was a trait that was required to manufacture the glucose testers. There were lots of tiny little pieces of electronic equipment and parts that needed to be soldered onto a small, printed circuit board. A terribly slow and exacting process which required an extremely steady hand and intense concentration.

There was also Simon, a person always interested in electronics and was working, at the time, at another electronics company in Brookvale. This was also close to the factory in Dee Why. Simon met Dad during his lunch break and immediately Dad was extremely impressed with his electronic knowledge and capabilities. Simon was also a key addition to the production of the glucose testers and, together with Mary, the two of them worked tirelessly and meticulously to ensure the entire process of making the glucose testers was achieved smoothly.

Then along came Jean. Jean was a good friend of Mary's and as Mary had been such an integral part of the business for so many years, she realised that Mum could not manage all the aspects of running the administration side of the business all by herself.

After a brief discussion between Mary and Mum, it was decided that Mary's friend Jean come in for a trial to help Mum with the packing of the testers. This was quite an important part of the business as it was extremely important that all the correct items were packed with the glucose testers. There was an important check list which needed to be followed directly and precisely to ensure that the glucose testers were sent out with the correct test strips. One test strip required to have the blood wiped off and the other test strip required to have the blood washed off. Putting the correct test strip into the box for postage or the courier was something that required 100% concentration. If the wrong strips were supplied with the tester, it would mean that the diabetic receiving the machine would be using the wrong strip, something that most certainly could have resulted in an extremely detrimental outcome.

After a couple of days of working with Mum, Jean became another important addition to our growing business family. Her accuracy with what she packed into the little cases that the machines were supplied in was beyond remarkable. She would check, double check, and check once more to make sure that every single item that needed to be sent out with the glucose tester was in the case. This did not only mean the strips that were supplied with the machines were correct but also that each case had a power transformer, a finger pricker, as well as an easy to read and very straight forward instruction manual. This all needed to be packed carefully with bubble wrap to ensure the glucose testers would not be damaged during transit.

It was also extremely important that the serial number of each machine was sent to the correct person so yet again Jean's job was that much more important. Jean carried out this job for many years and although it was hard work Jean found it very satisfying knowing that she never once, during the time she was with us, sent the wrong strips with a machine and with her fabulous packing, never once did a glucose tester arrive damaged.

We also had Nel working in our close-knit working environment. Nel worked very closely with Mary and Simon, she also helped them with production. Nel was another fabulous addition to our business and her work was very precise and her help was very appreciated by all of us as the orders were growing and the extra amount of glucose testers needing to be assembled was enormous.

Over the years, Mum and Dad did employ other people however some did not quite fit well with our tight knit "family" of employees. Therefore, our core staff all worked extremely hard to make sure the business never missed a beat.

The factory was also remarkably close to the post office, supermarkets, the newsagency, the bank, and the chemist. Absolutely everything we required was within a short walking distance. This made life easier for Mum when she needed to get groceries in a rush, post any mail and even pay bills.

As fantastic as the location was, the factory became much too small for Dad to continue manufacturing at such a large and rapid pace. Within a few months of the realisation that the factory was too small, we moved from the fish shop factory to a double story factory in Brookvale. We felt very posh as this factory had a board room. It had several offices, a large manufacturing room, a storeroom as well as his and hers toilets. It was on a corner block and once again the factory was in a very central location. We were there for many years until Dad realised that the rent being paid for the factory was paying the landlord's mortgage and as the business was continuing to grow, we also needed more room, yet again.

CHAPTER 20

# FACTORY PROGRESSION

Dad set out to buy a factory that was suitable for our needs. It became a nightmare to find something that fulfilled all his specific requirements that was also within budget. Thankfully, Dad was able to secure a small block of land that was affordable and in a great location.

The block of land was on the corner of two main roads which were connected to the very same bus route that our original factory had been located. The zoning of the property was spot on for Dad's requirements to build his own purpose-built factory.

We did continue to rent the factory in Brookvale as we could not cease operations at any time. The orders were coming through at a greater pace than ever, and Dad spent many months designing a factory that would fulfil every current need that he could have as the business grew.

Dad, together with Mum, worked tirelessly to not only keep up with manufacturing but also to finalise the plans of the new factory to be submitted and approved by the local council. Dad was also governed by council regulations in relation to the size of rooms, number of parking spaces required, as well as building height restrictions. A list that needed every little detail ticked off to perfection before council would approve it. My Dad's brain never stopped. He was happy with little sleep and would wake up every day with new thoughts and creative ideas.

Council quickly approved Dad's factory for construction to begin and the exciting part came when the little old house that had stood proud on the block was knocked down. Although, I must say, I am surprised the little old house needed to be knocked down, as it was almost falling over anyway. Shortly after Dad had purchased the block of land with the little old house, I took the opportunity to move in which allowed me to gain some sort of independence as I was not only living with Mum and Dad but also working with them.

It was a little weatherboard house with a high-pitched roof and a small but well covered veranda at the front. It had a stunning stone fireplace in the lounge room, which was certainly the centre piece of the room, together with two bedrooms off to the side of the long hallway which proudly staged the walkway through to the lounge room. The two bedrooms were extremely large, and the entire house had an extremely high ceiling which created a sense of space. It also presented itself with a beautifully detailed cornice around the ceiling.

The main bedroom also contained a stone fireplace. Although it was not as large as the one in the lounge room, it was certainly a lovely feature of that room. Every internal and external door was solid wood and there was even stained glass above the doors between each room. The little old house had the oldest carpet which I can honestly say was the original carpet which although old, it was immaculate and still in fantastic condition.

There was also a sunroom on the side of the house which adjoined the kitchen. In the mornings, this room was filled with natural light shining through the old, panelled stain glassed windows. This was lovely and warm in winter however during summer, the little old house's sunroom felt like a sauna.

The people that Dad bought it from used the little sunroom as a dining room. As you walked from the kitchen, through to the back of the house, you would enter a large concrete and brick laundry. It had an old concrete double sink which stood proud against one of the walls but certainly did not absorb the space. This room was also lit by the old glass louvred windows allowing the same light through that the sunroom offered.

Thankfully, in summer, the concrete and brick wall would keep the heat out. In winter, the laundry was absolutely freezing. Perfect in summer but the daunting thought of entering a cold laundry from a toasty warm lounge room with a fireplace was not very enjoyable. I have a feeling the house would have been over 60 years old when it was knocked down.

The land was perfectly level and was approximately 800 square metres in size. It had perfect access for cars and trucks and although it did not have curb and guttering, there were never any problems with flooding during heavy rain. It was such a shame that a little old house with so much charisma and charm was to be knocked down, something that sadly broke Dad's heart, however it was the only available and affordable land in the area that Dad could find to build his own, custom made and purpose-built factory.

After months of building, the factory was ready to move in to. It was a double story brick construction. There was a warehouse within which had a double story roller door, a kitchen, his and hers toilets both upstairs and down, as well as a very modern and welcoming front entrance. There were two separate offices together with a large manufacturing room. Access to the carpark was a concrete driveway and the truck access to the warehouse side of the factory was also concrete.

The small garden out the front was perfectly landscaped so the entire factory with its brown tone mottled bricks and a light brown roof looked very modern and impressive. Dad even created a small outdoor eating area for the staff. This was out the back in the very private open courtyard. It was also perfect in winter as the courtyard was protected from the wind, but the area was filled with winter sun, something that was extremely appreciated by our fabulous "family" staff members.

We were incredibly sad to leave the factory in Brookvale as we had been there for years however, we certainly didn't take very long to settle into our new factory. Even the staff felt at home in the brand-new place.

CHAPTER 21

# THE FACE OF THE BUSINESS

It was when we had the factory in Brookvale, I had completed high school, finished a 12-month secretarial course at Brookvale Technical College and had just got my very first full-time job working as a secretary and assistant to an accountant in Manly. I worked for the accountant for approximately 12 months and realised that Dad really needed help with the training and education of people using the glucose testers. I had been driving for a while at this stage and although Dad, over the years, had his own staff members helping him with visit to the hospitals, chemists, education centres and Endocrinologists for training in the use of the glucose testers.

It was now my turn to step up and help with a business I was the cause of. At the ripe old age of about seventeen, I thought it was important for me to be the one person that would drive to all the hospitals, chemists, doctors, education centres and be the educator of how to use the machines and how to calibrate them for accuracy. Accuracy was always important for the correct levels, as well as making sure that people were trained to put the correct amount of blood on the test strips.

I would travel to every corner of NSW to visit the hospitals and liaise with the Diabetic Educators. I would instruct the nursing staff in the hospitals how to use the glucose testers. I would also do night-time training for the shift workers so that every part of the nursing staff would either individually know how to use the tester properly or would be able to teach another staff member how to use it correctly. I did this for many years and would also travel to many other parts of Australia.

As the years went on, Mum had people contact her asking if they could be an agent for the business. This would mean that they looked after the state they were in. Mum and Dad would have specific requirements of the companies that asked to be an agent. It was extremely important that the people wanting to do this were reputable, reliable people and it was also important that not only Mum and Dad could rely on their product representation but also that of the diabetic requiring a new glucose tester.

Upon sourcing the appropriate representatives for the business, I would travel to their premises and train their staff how to use the glucose testers correctly. This was a time-consuming task as some of the agents had many staff members. I usually spent about a week with each company, making sure that after that time they were all competent and confident with themselves training people how to use the testers. I would always arrive on the Sunday to start a new week bright and early on the Monday morning and stay until the Friday. This time frame would also give the staff the time to ask any questions as the week went on. I did not want them to be overwhelmed with information and training and although the testers were extremely easy to use, it was extremely important that the people training new users needed to be one hundred percent sure they knew what they were doing.

During my time working with Dad, I met some beautiful caring people. They were so grateful, not only to Dad for his fantastic creation but also to me for being the one Dad created the glucose tester for. About seventy percent of the people that I would visit would graciously invite me to stay with them in their own homes. We did have a great repour with them so prior to me saying I would stay I felt assured and comfortable, in my mind, that I would be safe and well looked after. This is something that was also particularly important to Mum and Dad as being their only child it was of crucial importance to them both.

One advantage of me staying with these beautiful caring people was that they had diabetes in their lives in one way or another. That is why they were involved with either a Diabetes Australia branch or they were involved as a diabetic educator or a nurse. I even had an Endocrinologists sister ask me to stay with her in Lismore. These incredible people would always make sure I was comfortable and very well fed. Some would also do my washing if I were there any longer than a couple of days. To this day, I cannot thank them enough for their love and care, for the food, the accommodation but most of all for their support. Not only did they support me during the time I was with them, but they supported Mum and Dad during a massive part of our family's lives. During this period in my early life, I experienced many new adventures in different places throughout Australia and look back on this period of my life with fond memories.

Dad's business was a constantly evolving creation that was not showing any sign of slowing down. We were supplying glucose testers all over the world and to some extremely influential people which included a renowned Russian politician. His secretary came to Australia and collected a glucose tester from Dad's factory. I really do believe that it was at this time that Dad realised that he had created an absolute phenomenon, not only in Australia but throughout the world.

It was at this time that Dad was awarded the government contract to supply glucose testers to hospitals around Australia. Together with this contract we also obtained the contract for the Department of Veterans Affairs which was associated with Concord Hospital. This dramatically created an uptake of orders and Australian BIO Transducers was inundated with orders.

I can honestly say that over the years our glucose testers were a very patient friendly and widely embraced piece of medical equipment in an extremely large percentage of hospitals around the country, and indeed around the world. I have a feeling that we could find a hospital name starting with each letter of the alphabet. It went from Armidale, Brisbane, Canberra, Dubbo, Eveleigh, Forbes, Gunnedah, Hornsby, Ipswich, John Hunter, and the list continues. All the major hospitals around Australia had Dad's glucose testers, together with most of the smaller hospitals whether they were public or private.

CHAPTER 22

# ANOTHER AUSTRALIAN FIRST

Within a short period of time, Dad was aware that the glucose testers were a one-off cost. He had been made aware that the imported test strips used for home blood glucose testing was seeing millions of Australian dollars, per year, go overseas to the multi-national companies for their supply of strips.

There were, at this stage, other glucose testers available and as it only takes a few small changes to create a new product, the multi nationals had created their own brand of designs. They then used their own machines to negotiate supply with the hospitals and doctors to promote and use their brand of machines and strips. This in turn meant that the consumable product, being the blood test strip, would be used constantly by those that purchased the multi-national brand glucose tester. Only their strips worked with their testers. Thus, ensuring ongoing sales.

Dad, being concerned that the overseas companies were making a massive amount of money from their test strips, decided to work on developing an Australian made blood glucose strip that would be for use with his glucose testers only. This would mean that an extremely large amount of money would be kept in Australia's "hands", and he felt this would help the Australian economy. The amazing thing about my Dad was that he never once thought of himself, but always about other people and Australia's financial savings.

Dad had a friend who was a bio chemist at a Sydney University and together they decided they should work on developing a blood glucose test strip. Together they worked around the clock, in between their own daily lives, to produce the world's first Australian blood glucose strip. Dad had even met two people who were involved in making industrial refrigerators and ovens and it was these two men that created an oven to produce the strips at the necessary temperature without any heat variation. We still, today, have this oven in our shed.

After several months of creating the test strip, it was approved for accuracy. Dad was extremely happy as he now had a strip specifically for his own glucose testers. This meant that the profits from his strips would be used for research within the Australian diabetic system or to put towards creating more technology for faster testing as well as towards manufacturing smaller testers.

Within months of Dad creating an Australian blood glucose testing strip, he was awarded with the government contract to supply the hospitals with our "Easy scan" test strips. This simply meant that all the government hospitals around Australia would use Dad's glucose testers and the "Easy scan" test strips. This was a remarkable achievement as this would prevent millions of Australian dollars, every year, leaving Australia and being pocketed by the multinational companies, solely on the sales of the glucose test strips.

The glucose strips were yet another brilliant and amazing development created by my exceptionally talented and sensational Dad. His team had not only developed the strips, but they had made the cutting machine and the oven to manufacture them. They also sourced the most affordable and perfect packaging for the strips.

It was within a few weeks of Dad receiving the news about the government contract for the strips that I informed the very first person about our strips due release date. This information was given to a Diabetic Educator at one of the large hospitals in NSW. This education centre was one of the largest we dealt with, and I was delighted to be able to share the information with such a supportive Educator.

This was massive news for the diabetes groups, not only in Australia but also around the world as Dad's strips were extremely affordable and readily available due to the fabulous team of people that helped Dad's business manufacture at an amazing rate.

Dad was delighted with his strips as he understood that this would now allow Australia's wealth to increase by saving such a massive amount of money to be given to an overseas economy. Dad saw it as money for Australian infrastructure, medicine, as well as research and development. The research and development part was something my Dad was extremely passionate about. Dad was yet again incredibly grateful that he was able to achieve a major money saving consumable product that was extremely important in the life of people living with diabetes.

# CHAPTER 23

# THE BEGINNING OF THE END

The word about our release date for the strip spread extremely quickly and within a couple of hours of the news being released, the big boss of one of the multi-national companies contacted Dad by phone and told him in no uncertain terms that if Dad was to release his strip, even initially in Australia, that he would put Dad out of business within six months of release.

My Dad was never one to give into harsh wording or threats and amazingly handled the phone call with a kind, professional response that basically suggested that he was not going to be intimidated by a man that thought he was bigger and much better than my Dad. After all, my Dad was the one that had created the entire affordable home testing system. He was also a man that was very humble and never blew his own trumpet at his success.

The strips were released, and Dad was determined not to let multi-national companies take his business from him and he continued, with all the help possible from Mum and myself, the employees together with our family and friends.

Within a few months, Mum and Dad were noticing that the sales of the glucose testers were diminishing. As I was still visiting the hospitals and education centres around Australia, particularly Sydney hospitals, I was also aware that the usual glucose testers were being replaced very rapidly with the multi-national company's new model testers. Initially I did not think too much about it and did my usual checks to make sure our glucose testers were working correctly and double checking the testers were cleaned properly.

It was also important that I taught any new additions to the team of educators and or nurses. I would visit each clinic about every eight weeks or so and it was this next visit to several clinics and hospital wards, including emergency departments, that I noticed none of our machines were available for me to check. As I had dealt with so many of the staff at the hospitals and education centres for many years, I approached the head of each department and asked where my Dad's glucose testers were. Sadly, most of the people that I dealt with were extremely heartbroken to inform me that a multinational company had replaced all the glucose testers in not only the wards and emergency but also all the glucose testers in the education centres.

This was a move that my poor Mum and Dad could not contend with or compete with. Although Dad had only just released his glucose testing strip, he could not financially replace all the hospital equipment with his own testers. Dad was fully aware that the reason for the move made by the multinational company was purely to make sure that their own test strips were not removed by using our machines and our Australian made glucose strips. After all, the glucose test strips were the consumable product. Millions of dollars were being spent every year on the overseas test strips in Australia alone, so Dad's strip was therefore a major threat to the multinational companies.

The fact was that the industry of glucose testing, not only Australia but the world, was large enough for any number of companies to operate successfully. Unfortunately, my Dad's extremely affordable glucose test strip was a very alarming threat to the multinational's. Basically, they needed to get Dad out of the diabetes environment for them to not be affected by their glucose strip sales that were to either fall or drop off altogether.

As the months went by, Mum and Dad were starting to see that our remarkably successful little business was being greatly affected by what the multinational companies were offering. They were giving away free glucose testers to hospitals, both public and private, medical centres, and chemists and this was purely to eliminate any of Dad's machines being out in the society of diabetics.

This basically meant that Dad's new strip would be useless in the market and with a glucose testing strip, as it was the only consumable product that created the multi millions of dollars being obtained not only in Australia but world-wide. The multinationals had a game plan and sadly, as the big boss of one of the multinational companies had warned my Dad, releasing Dad's strip would put Dad out of business within six months.

Within a few months, Dad's extremely successful business had gone from a remarkable influx of orders for new machines to a saddening manufacturing reduction as the sales were no longer coming in. After a short period of time, Dad was reluctantly forced to ask some of his very loyal and supportive staff to leave. He did require some help with continuing the business with a few repairs coming in from time to time as by this stage, some of the very first machines were coming in for either intense cleaning or reconditioning of the testers for their next ten years of use. With all the machines out in the worldwide market, it was amazing that most repairs were purely from people dropping them, or simply being a little heavy handed with battery replacement or cleaning.

Mum and Dad still operated the business as they needed to be on hand for anything anyone required. Sadly, the cost of keeping the purpose-built factory that Dad had put so much time, effort, and passion into building and designing was beyond a cost that Mum and Dad were able to continue to afford.

They were left with the heartbreaking decision to sell the factory. They were able to pay their mortgage off on the factory and then had to make the decision to rent a much smaller factory which was literally around the corner from Dad's purpose-built factory. They made this decision as the location of the factory was always especially important to both Mum and Dad. They both considered the access and location for anyone who could not drive so therefore being close to a bus stop was a necessary factor.

The new factory, which was one of four in the complex, was close to the factory we had just vacated. It was situated around the corner from the previous location which meant anyone needing or wanting to visit the new premises would know exactly where to go.

## CHAPTER 24

# MY NEWFOUND ROLE

I was basically forced to leave the business in a role that meant so much to me for so many years. The sales had ceased to a point where the bills were still coming into the factory yet the funds from the sales was virtually non-existent at his stage. Although I worked for Dad for many years at such a young age, I had previously worked as an accountant's secretary. It was not the thought of working for someone else that concerned me, it was simply the fact that I was so very passionate about what our family had created, and we worked together so well for so long. I was heartbroken to watch us lose something that had been created by my very amazing and successful Dad, all for his love of helping me live a better life.

I was living out of home at this stage, so it was imperative that I find a job. I had bills to pay as I had bought myself a unit several years before the business ended. I had a mortgage, bills and a car which did not come cheap so I needed to find something as close to home as I could and something that I was passionate about. As I had previously worked for an accountant, I had the option of returning to that type of work. I did enjoy working as a secretary so something along the same lines was important to me. This was also in the day where jobs were advertised in the local paper, unlike on the internet or an employment agency website. Thankfully, our local newspaper was quite a large publication, so I had pages and pages of jobs to apply for. I had also made the decision to try to find a job in medicine, either at a pharmacy or a doctor's surgery.

My very first job during my years at school, was a Thursday night job cleaning shelves, unpacking stock, and serving customers in our local chemist. I was there many years and really enjoyed the interaction with the customers. I remember my first customer was a young man asking me for help with his choice of condoms. I was gobsmacked and flustered as I had absolutely no idea how to handle this customer. I was also entirely unsure of what to say to him. I was embarrassed however I was as professional as I could be and hopefully assisted him with his purchase. As the months went on, I realised that I thoroughly enjoyed speaking with the people who were unwell, and I constantly tried to help them feel better simply by listening to their pains and ailments. I was there for many years and was at that point I began my secretarial course at Brookvale Technical College.

With my role in Dad's business, I spent many hours working in a hospital environment, and I realised that it was important for me to follow my passion of working with people in the medical industry. My compassion for the unwell helped with the decision that made me apply for a medical receptionist job at Cremorne just north of Sydney. I had never had any problems speaking with people and nerves were never a concern to me when applying for a job, so I was quite confident after my contact with the doctor requiring a receptionist. I met with him the following day and started within a few days later. It was a job share situation of four days a week. I was also required if the other receptionist was sick or on holidays.

Within a few weeks, I found my feet and really enjoyed my work as a medical receptionist. This was before the time of computers and everything that was carried out was hard copy paperwork and a card system for patient's records. It did involve a lot of paperwork and being a fully trained secretary, this is something I enjoyed and together with the other receptionist, we kept the surgery running like clockwork. The surgery was open six days a week, so if I was required for two or three weeks at a time, I was totally exhausted by the end. We started at 8.30 and finished at 6pm so it was a massive day. Thankfully, we had a good break during each day so I could go to the bank, and the post office. This would give me time to stretch my legs and clear my head. We had many food options around the Cremorne area although it was expensive. I generally chose to take may own lunch, often, and we thankfully had a fantastic lunchroom which had a table for six people. It also offered a microwave oven, a sandwich toaster, a large fridge and was always, at lunch time, bathed in beautiful sunshine.

I particularly enjoyed getting to know the patients. They had been patients for many years before I started at the surgery, but it was their welcoming and caring nature that helped me settle in very quickly and get to know them very well. I would joke with them, assist them, and enjoy our conversations. I even got to know their voices when they called to make an appointment. They would say "Lisa?" when I answered the phone and I would know approximately half of the patients' voices, without them saying anything else.

I held this position for many years and, also totally embraced the friendship and love that I found with the other professionals' and receptionists' who also shared the building. There were two dentists within the surgery and over the years I also got to know the dentists' patients and thoroughly enjoyed their company during their visit to a dentist. Certainly not something that anyone enjoys however the dentists' receptionists', and I would help pass their stressful waiting time by laughing and joking with them, obviously in between our work time.

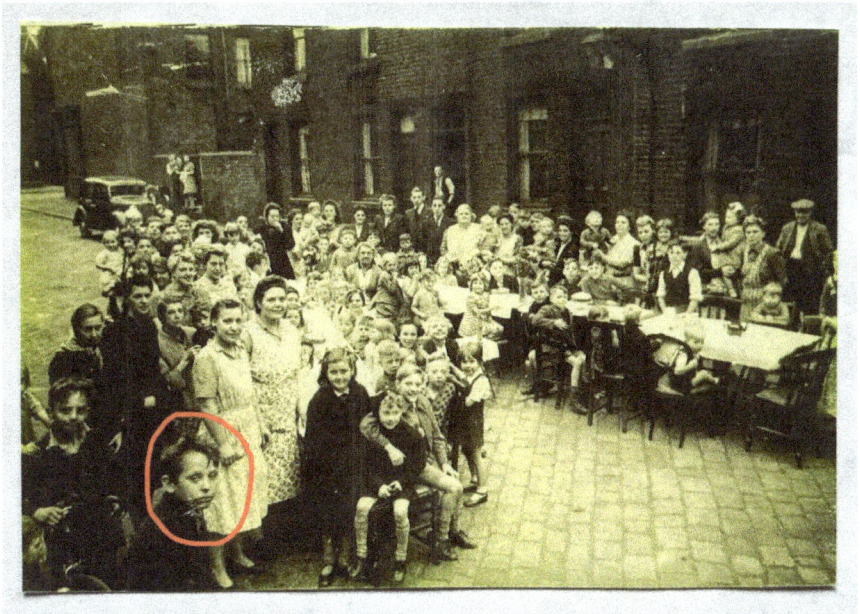

*Dad at the VE-day local area celebration*

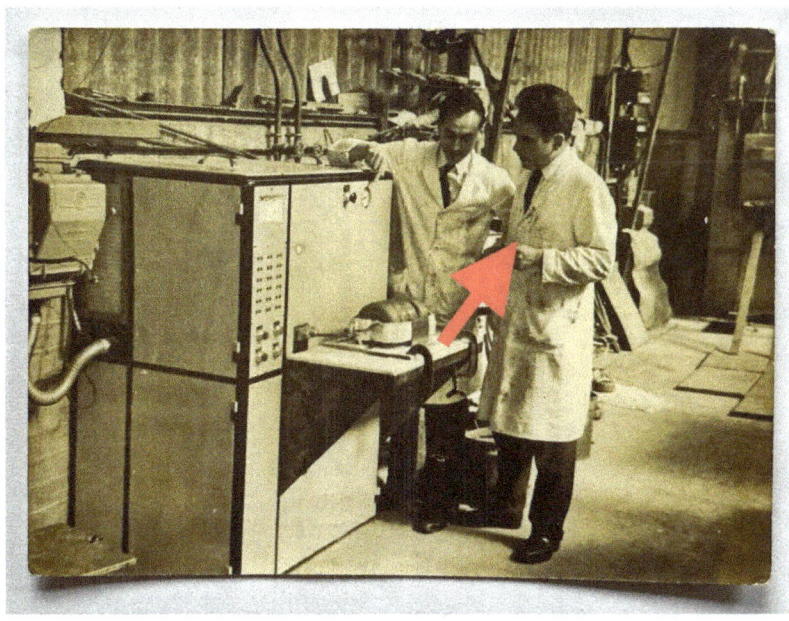

*Magnetic Machine made by Dad*

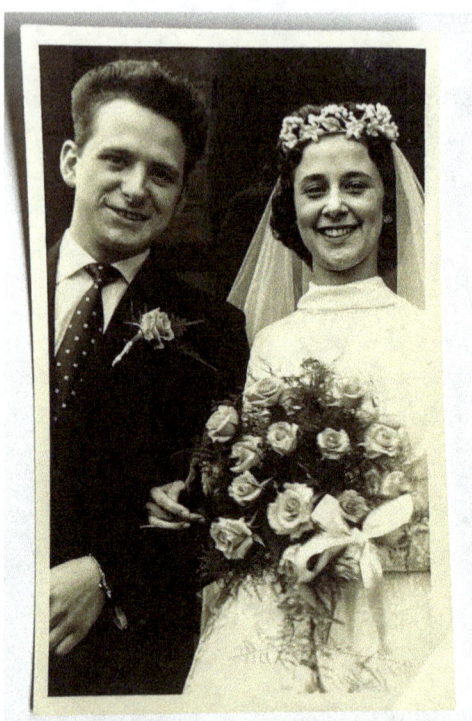

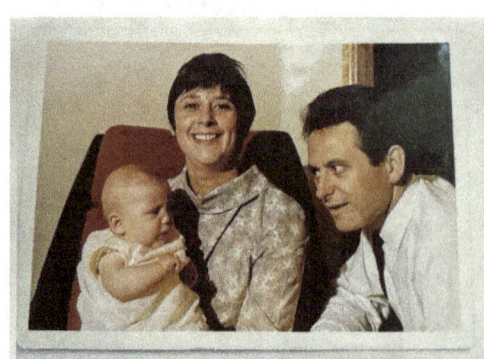

*Mum, Dad and myself 1967*

*Mum and Dad's wedding 1957*

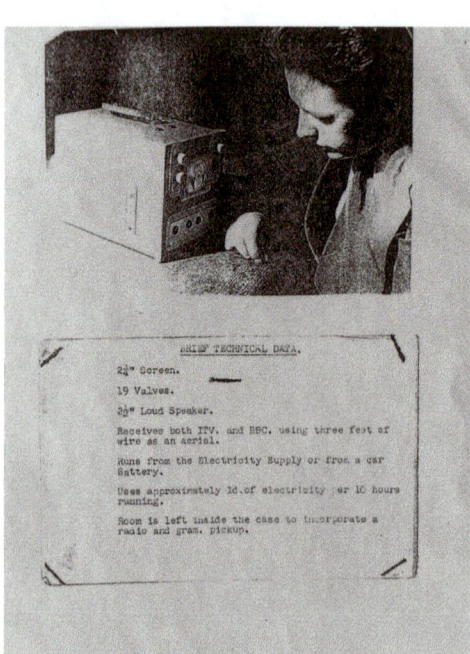

*Miniature tv made by Dad*

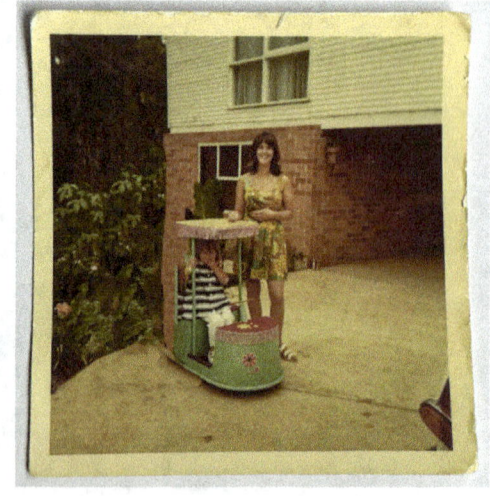

*My little car made for me by Dad 1970*

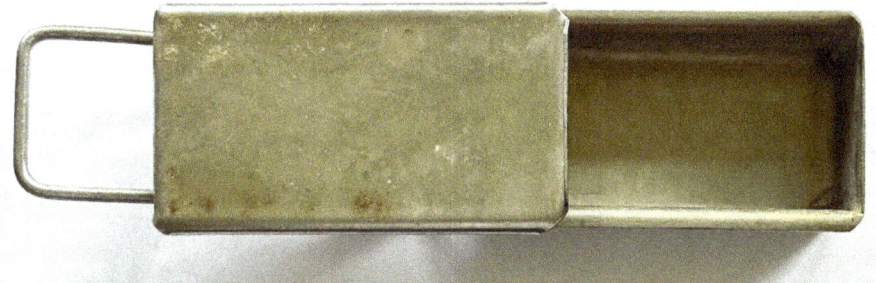

*My needle sterilizer made by my godfather*

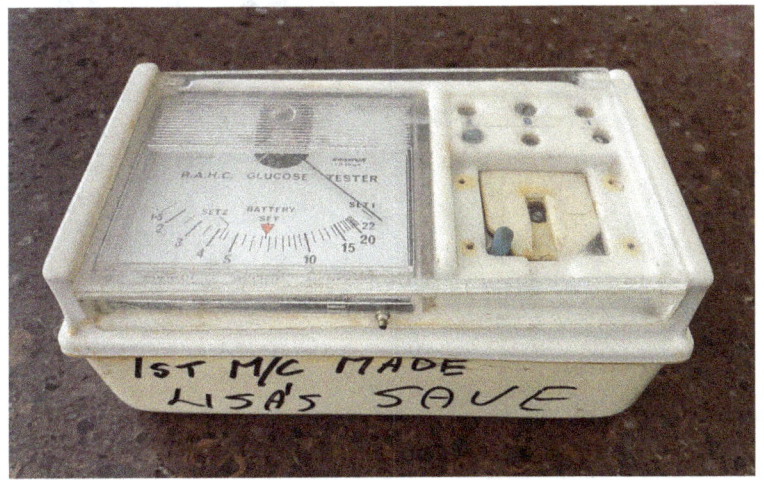

*The very first machine made for me 1978*

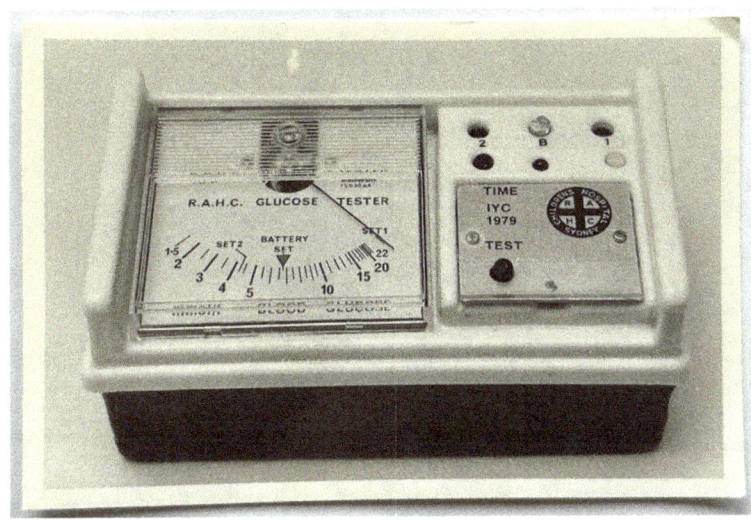

*RAHC model glucose tester*

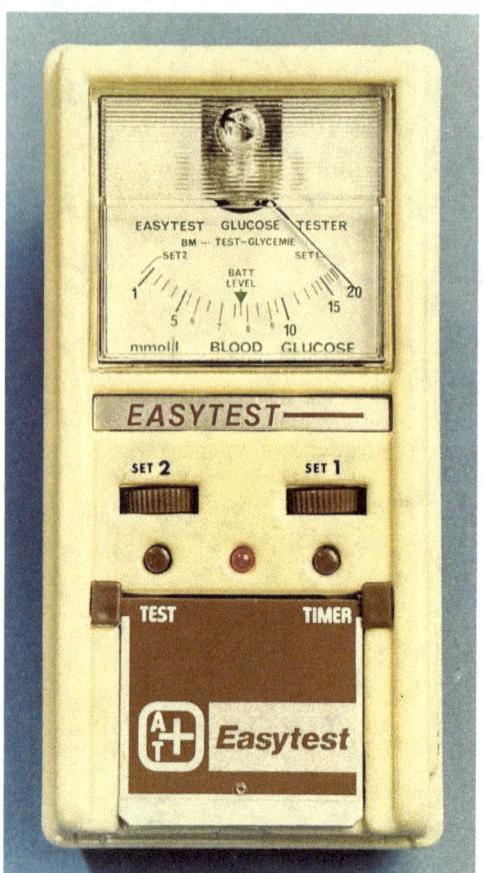

*Easytest model glucose tester*

*Glucotest 4000 model glucose tester*

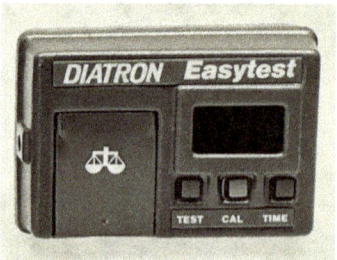

*Diatron model glucose tester*

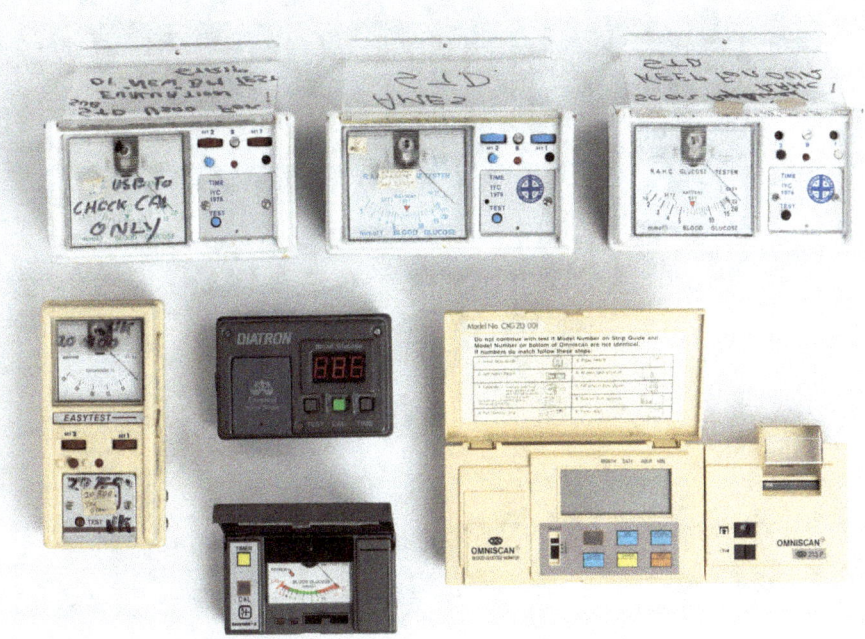

*Various models of glucose testers*
*Powerhouse Museum - Gift of Audrey Clark - Photographer Belinda Christie*

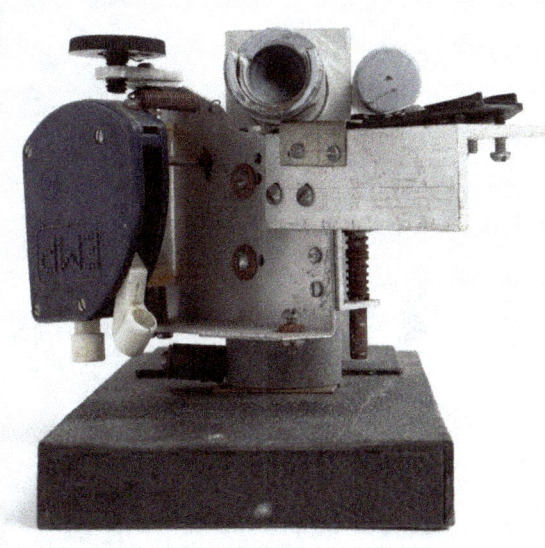

*Finger pricker prototype for the blind*
*Powerhouse Museum - Gift of Audrey Clark - Photographer Belinda Christie*

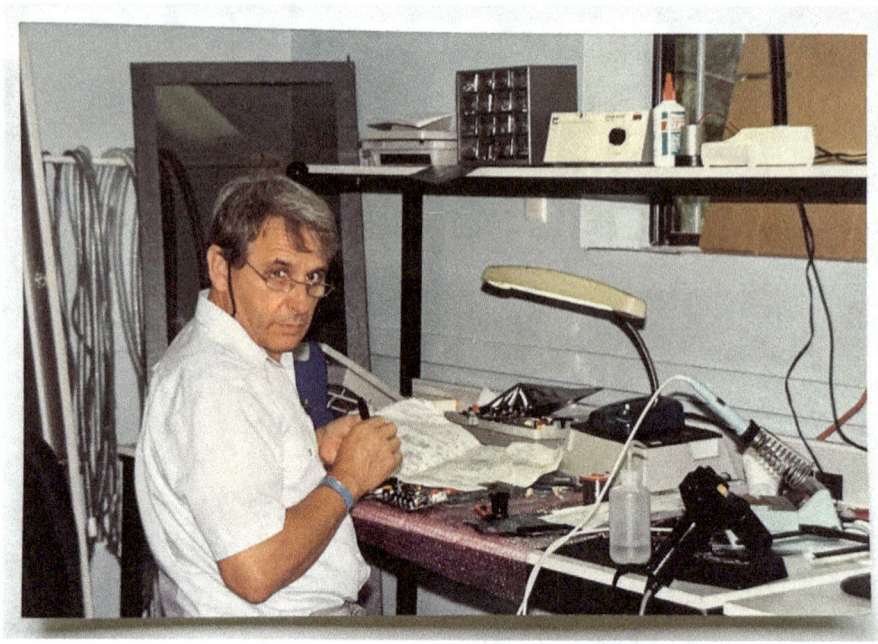

*Dad in his elements at his work bench*

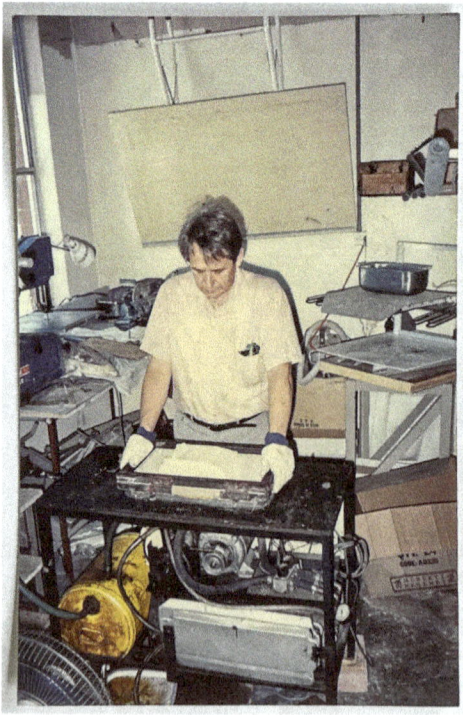

*Vacuum former designed and built by Dad to vacuum form cases for glucose tester*

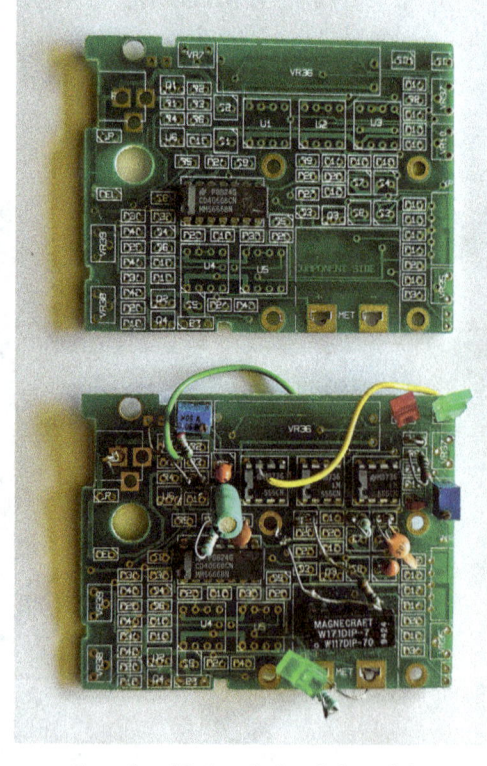

*Sample of Printed circuit board for glucose tester*

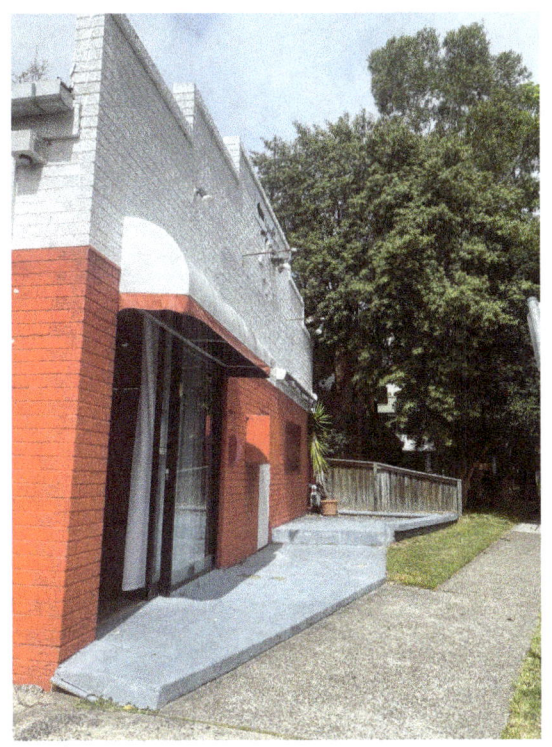

*First factory Dee Why in front of fish shop*

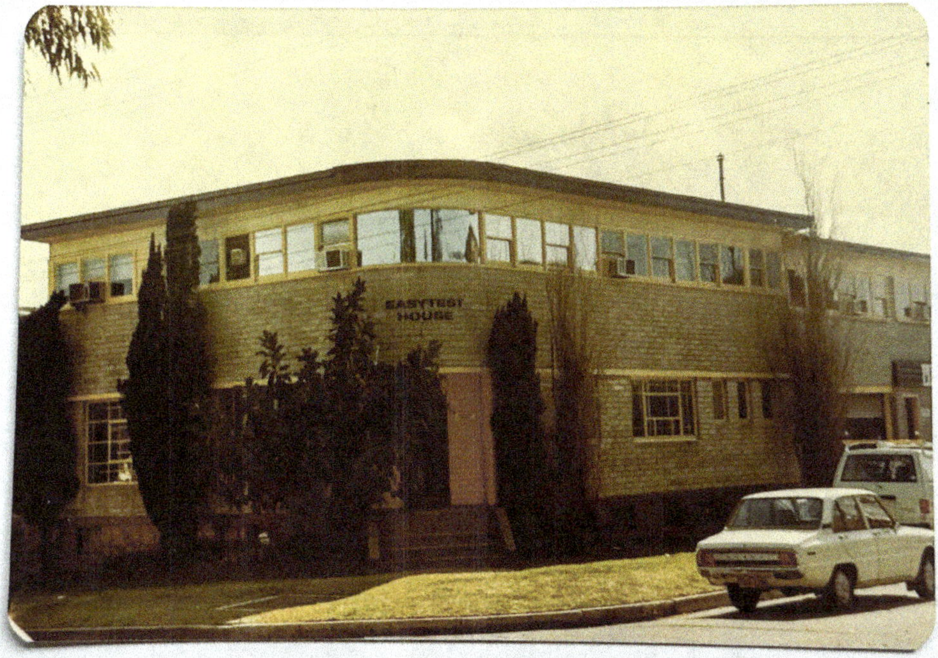

*Easytest House*

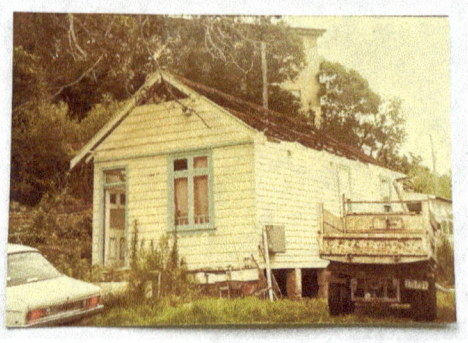

*Old house on the land chosen for the new factory construction*

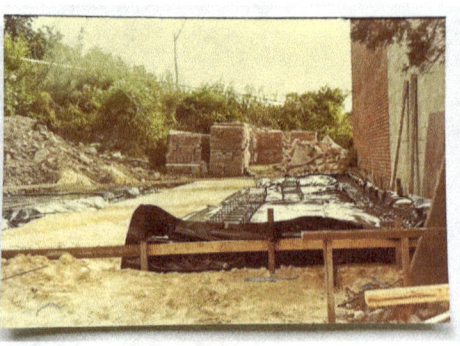

*Factory construction*

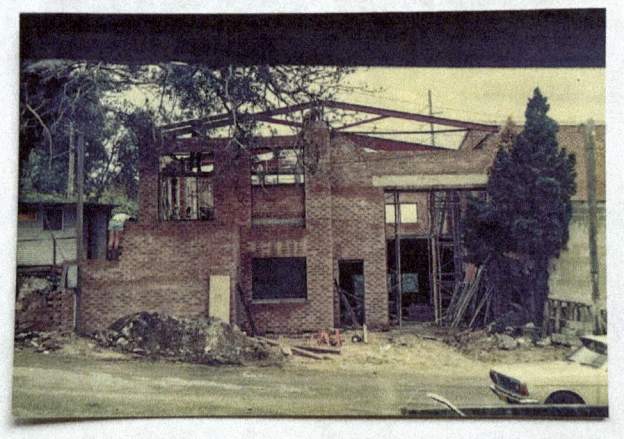

*Factory construction*

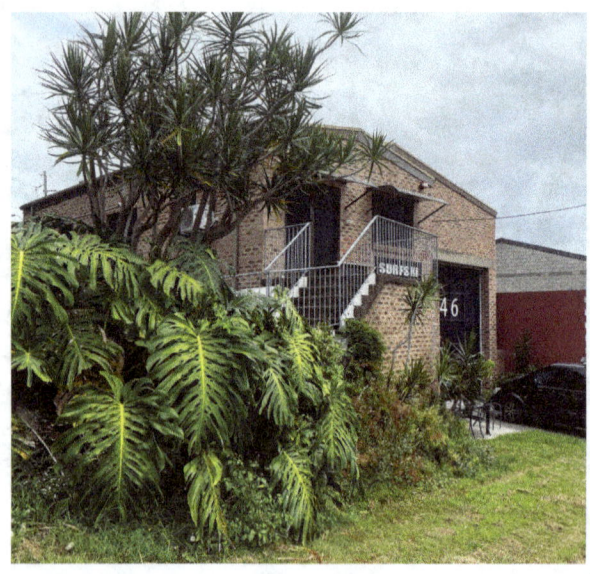

*Completed purpose built factory*

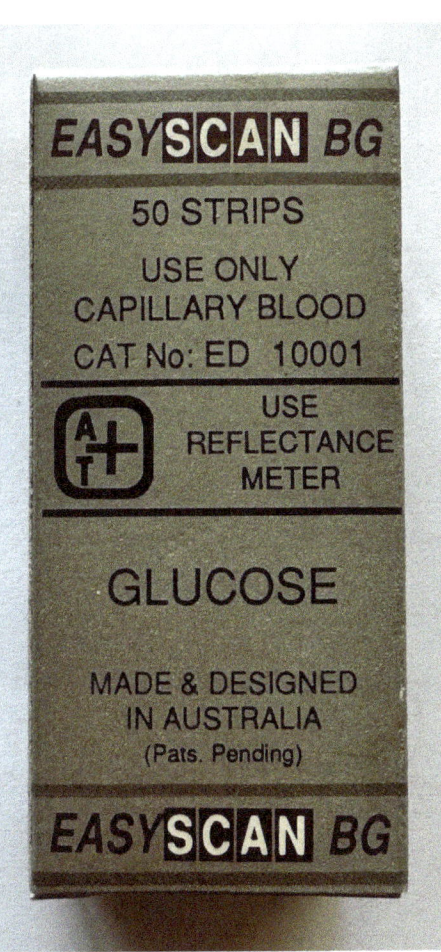

Dads Australian made test strips

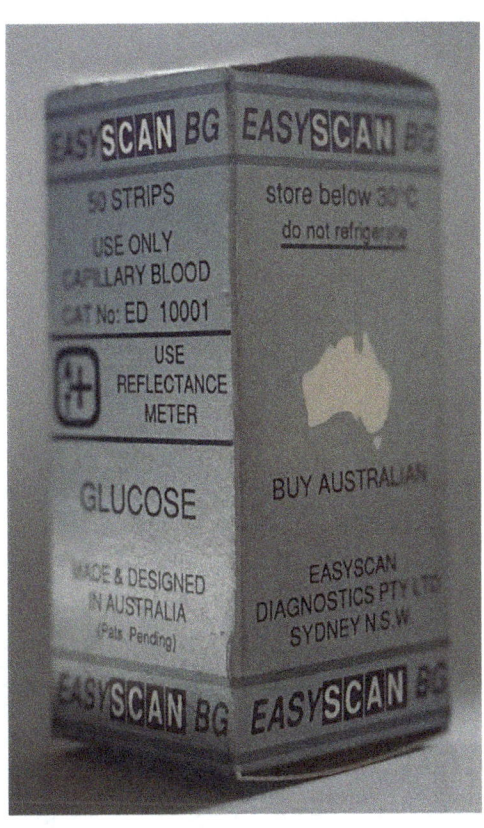

Dads Australian made test strips

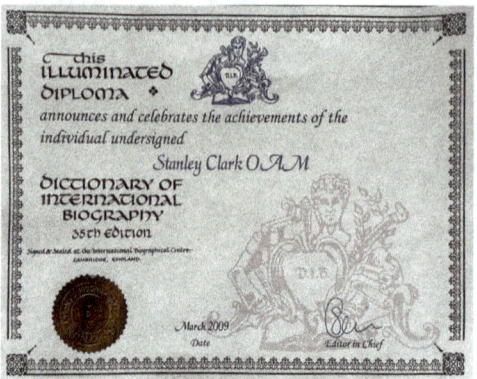

*Certificate*

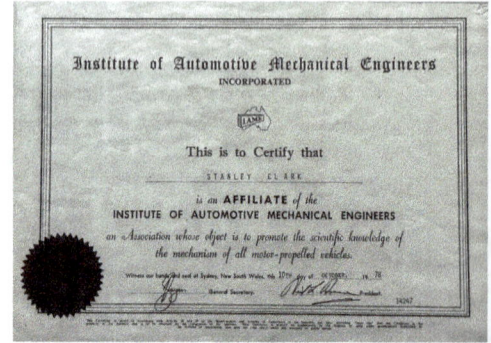

*Automotive Institute Award*

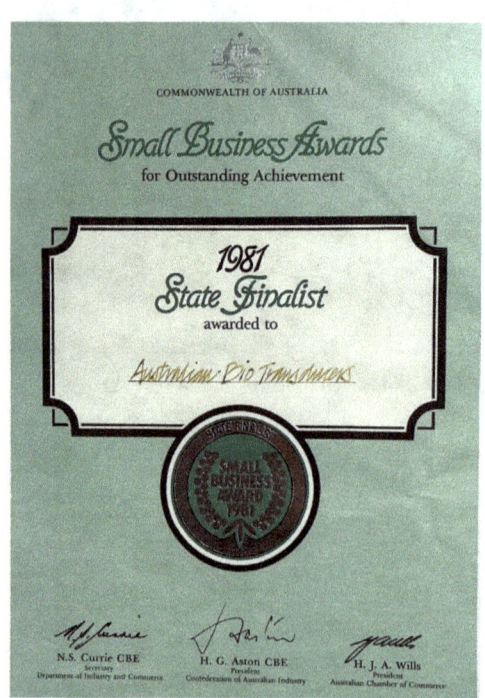

*Small Business Award*

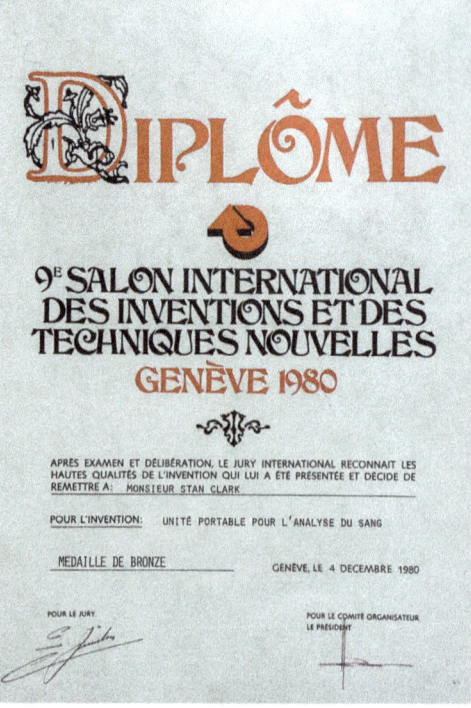

*Diplome*

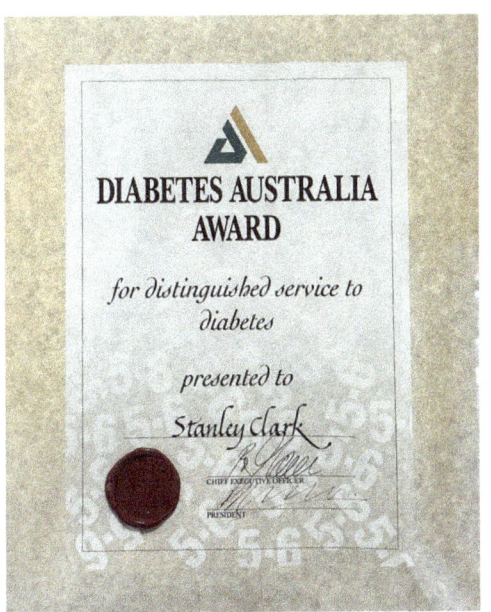

Diabetes Australia Award

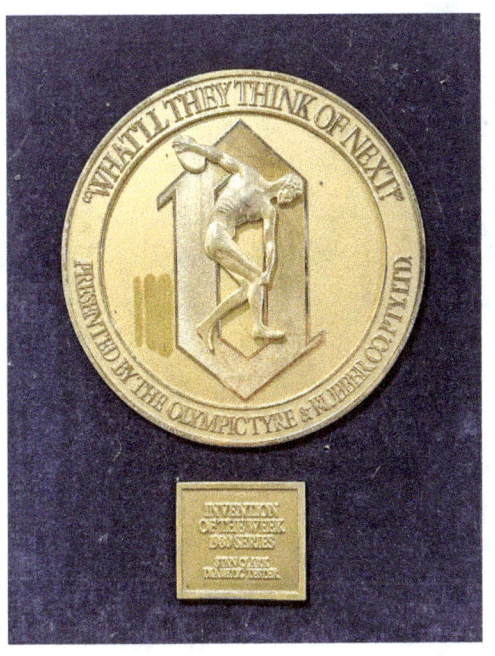

What'll They Think of Next Award

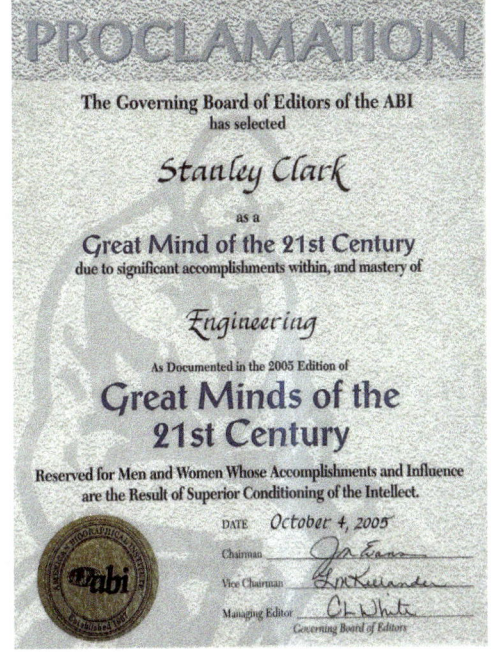

Great Minds of the 21st Century

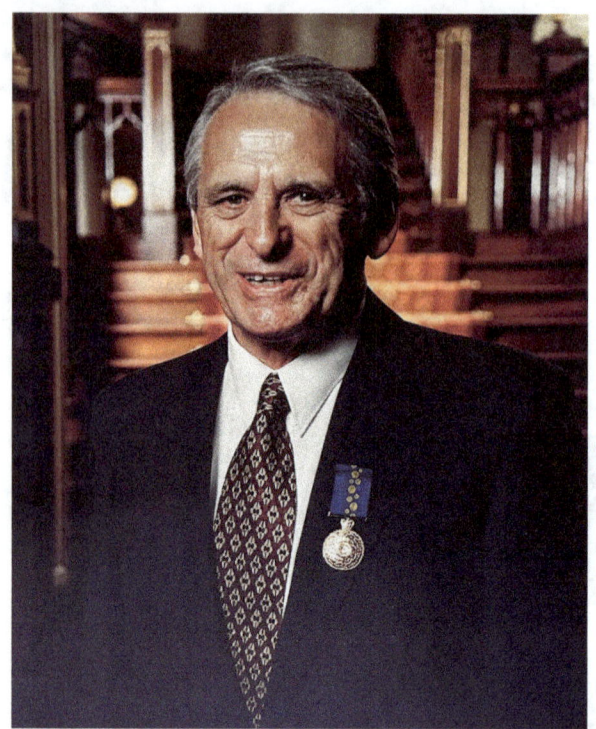

*Dad OAM*

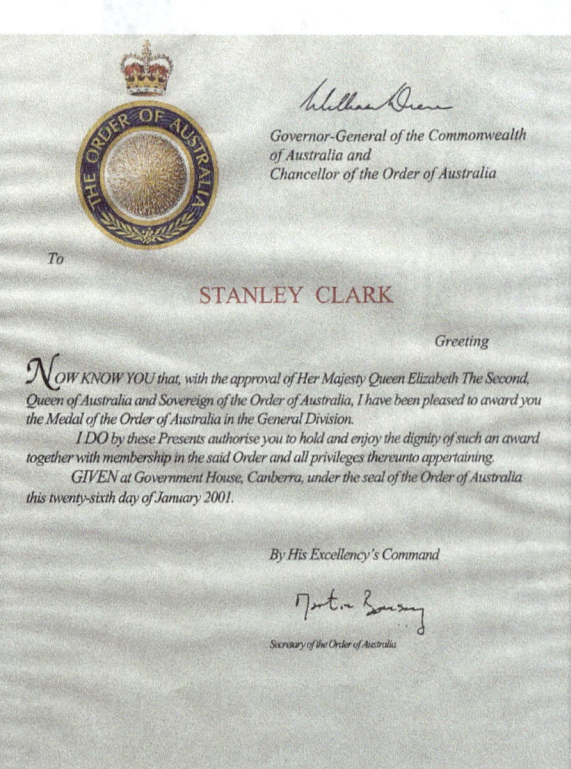

*Order of Australia*

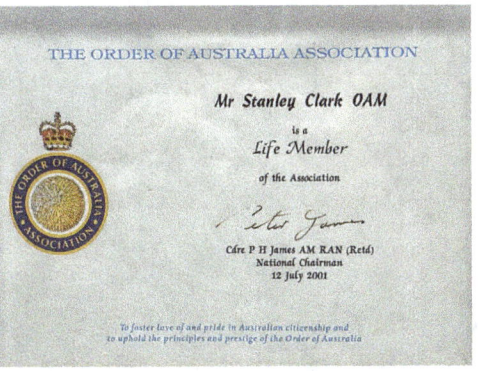

Order of Australia life member Certificate

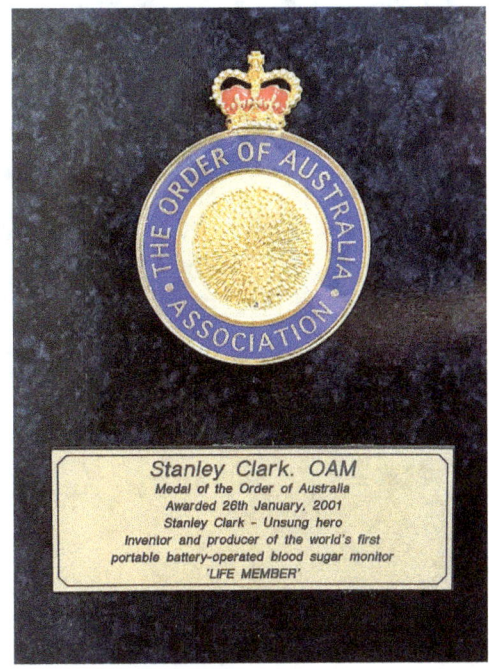

Order of Australia

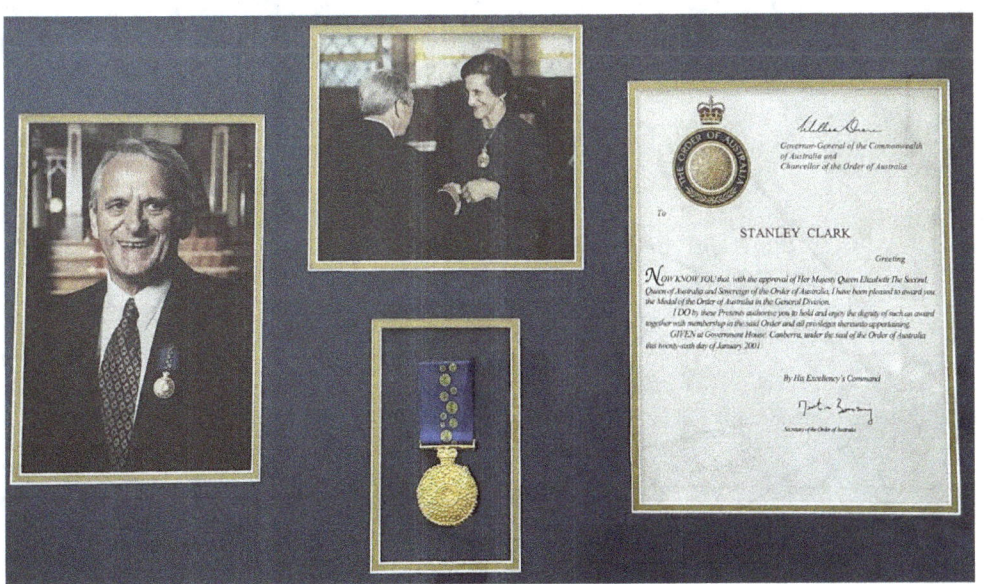

*A very proud moment*

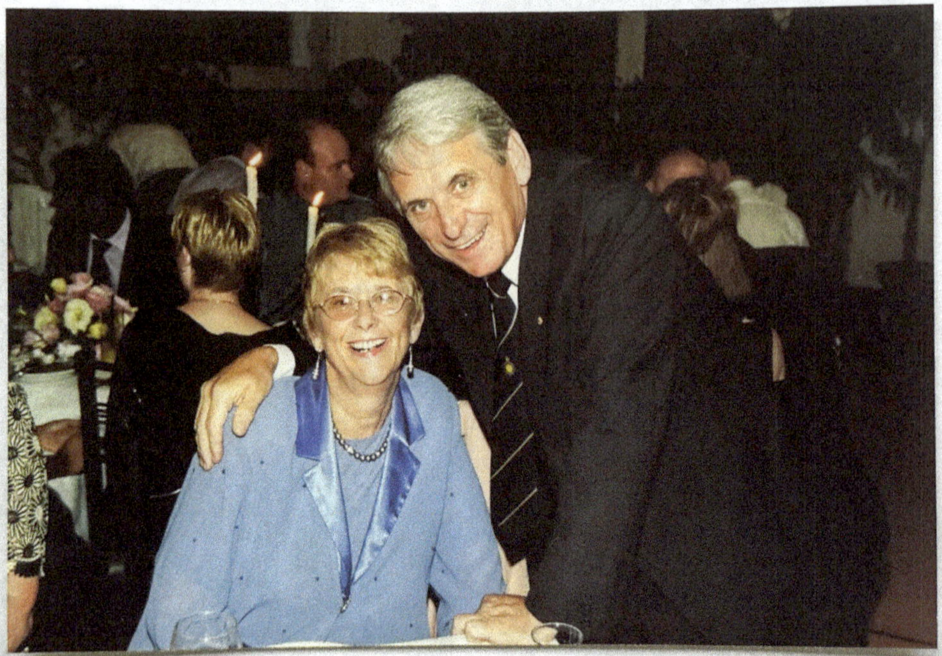

*Mum and Dad*

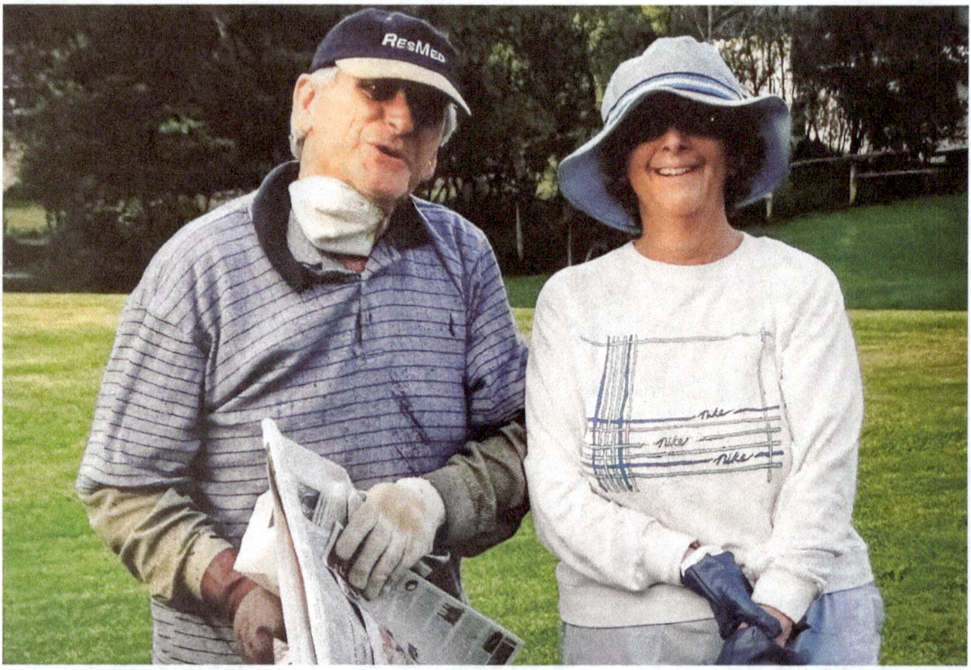

*Mum and dad in their early retirement*

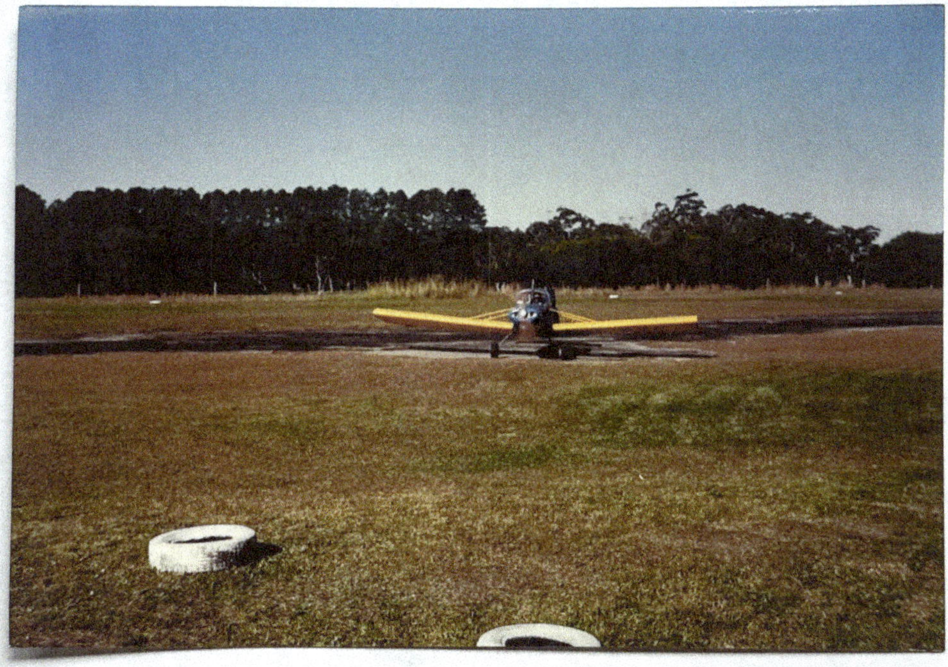

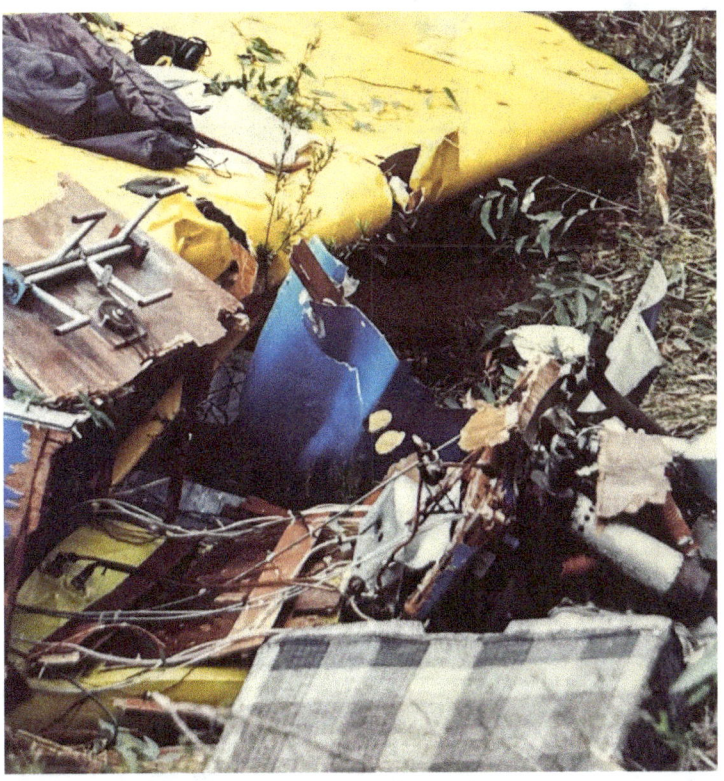

*Dad's plane prior to takeoff*

*Plane crash wreckage*

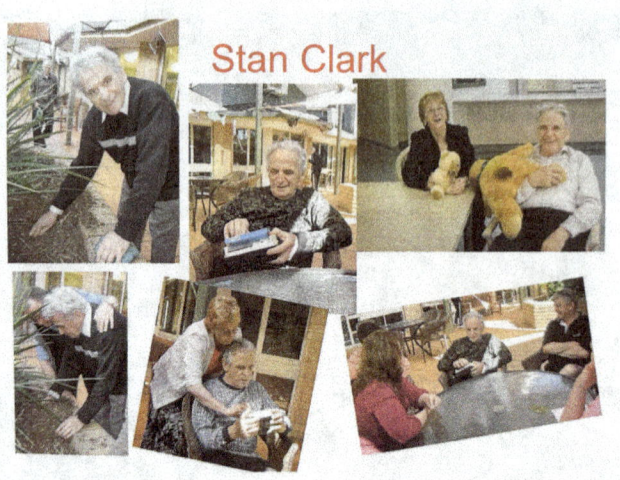

*Dad enjoying a memory of his great invention*

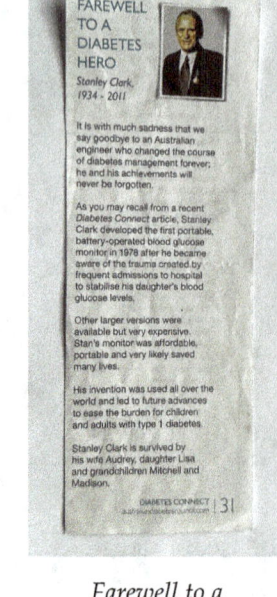

*Farewell to a Diabetes Hero*

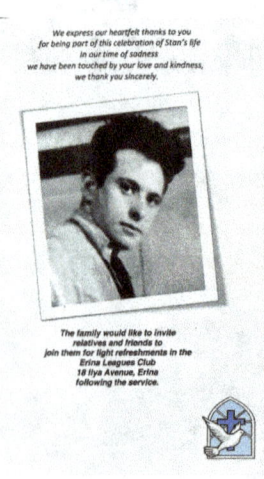
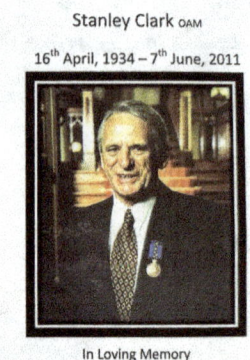

*Order of Service Dad's funeral*

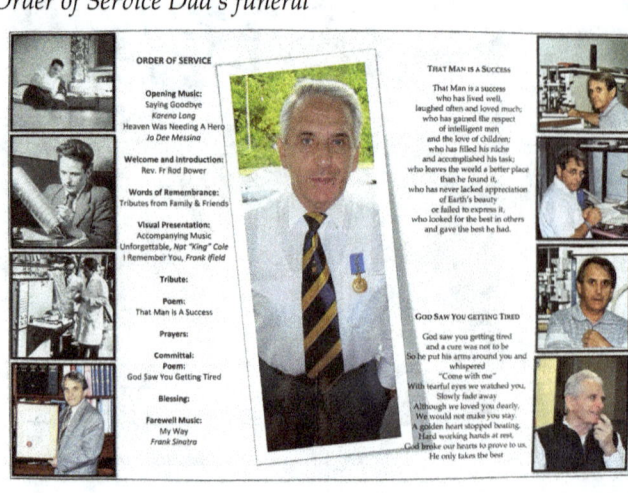

Live your life | Diabetes NSW

This certificate is presented to

**Lisa Harris**

In recognition of your appointment as

**Diabetes NSW Ambassador**

14 November 2014

Dr Neville Howard
President
Diabetes NSW

Sturt Eastwood
Chief Executive Officer
Diabetes NSW

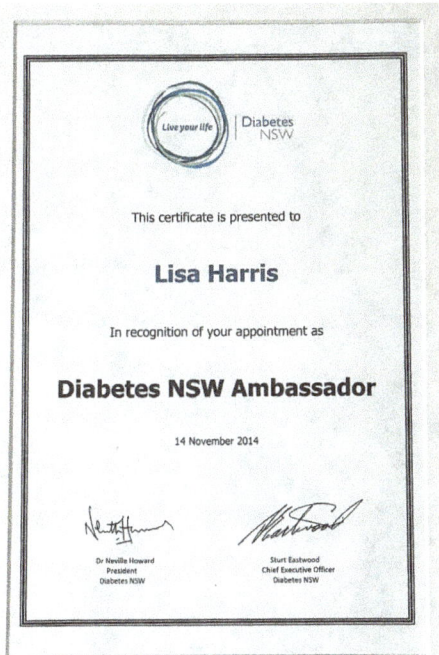

*Lisa Harris (Clark) Ambassador*

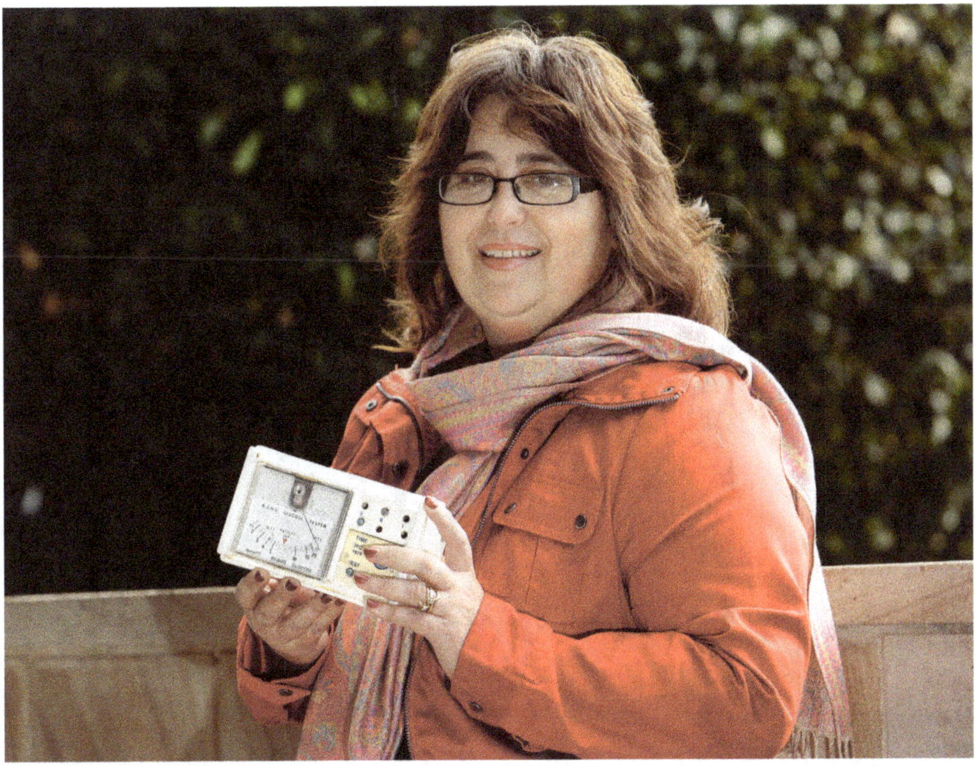

*Proudly holding my very first home blood glucose tester*
*Photographer Waide Maquire/Newspix*

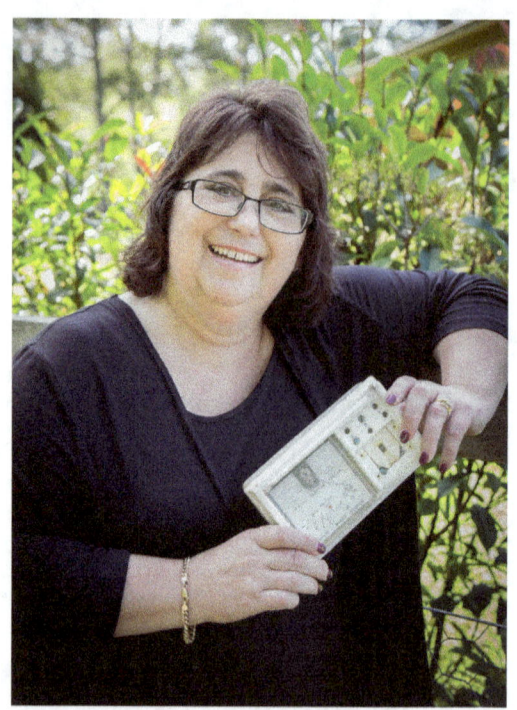

2021
*Hannah Rachael Photography*

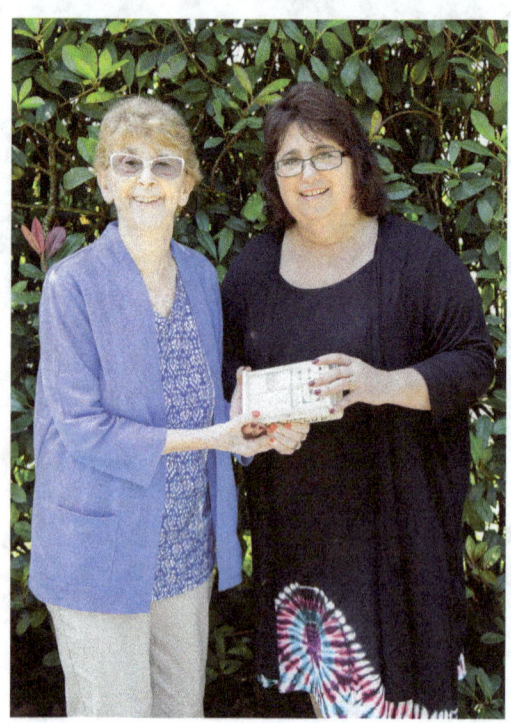

*A proud moment with my mum*
*Hannah Rachael Photography*

# CHAPTER 25

# A NEW YET COMPLICATED BEGINNING

During my time working at the surgery, I became pregnant with my first child. Just married and looking forward to my new arrival, I decided to continue working throughout my pregnancy which certainly made it easy for me when my routine blood tests were required. I had constant contact with the pathology company as we would receive urgent blood results via phone. Other results were delivered by the blood courier during their daily visit for collection of blood samples.

I remember one afternoon in particular, the pathologist rang and asked if he could speak with the doctor. They would always inform me of the patients name so I could pass this on to the doctor when transferring the call. I asked a couple of times and their response to this was that this test result is confidential.

The call had come through prior to the doctor returning from his house calls so I told the pathologist that I would have the doctor return his call as soon as possible. I was sitting at the reception desk as the call was made and was always aware that the surgery door would normally remain open until the first afternoon patient entered the room. It was a routine that over the years I was so used to, a routine that never changed. Even during important and urgent contact with any medical professional, the surgery door would remain open, and I was always aware of any conversation the GP was having.

After the call was made, I was aware that the doctor had come to the door between the surgery and the reception desk to close it. Although I thought it was a little strange and not his normal routine that he had always followed, I just thought it may have been a private result regarding one of the doctor's friends or family members, so I did not give it another thought. After about a five-minute phone call, the doctor asked me if he could have an outside line. Normally, he would just ask me to contact whoever he needed or wanted to speak with, once again, another routine that was quite different from the normal everyday routine we were so used to at the surgery.

The call, which was made by the doctor himself, lasted again, approximately five minutes. It was not unusual for a call to last this length of time so yet again; I did not think too much of it. I simply thought that I would be told of what was going on once the doctor was ready to discuss it with me. We had many conversations about the medical plan of all patients, as it was better for me to have some basic understanding of any requirements necessary for their care. I was then able to assist in any way possible to make sure the patient received the best care both within and outside the surgery.

The afternoon continued like any other normal afternoon however, it worked out that the last two appointments were cancelled so I was thinking to myself, maybe I can go home early. After all, I was 32 weeks pregnant. Thankfully, I was always able to take the weight off my feet whenever I needed to. The patients were fully aware of my pregnancy and were absolutely delighted for me. Most of them knew that I had diabetes and that my Dad had created the world's first home blood glucose tester. This fact is something that many of the patients were very passionate about as they also had diabetes. Both type 1 and type 2 diabetes patients would speak with me often and to know that I, as a diabetic, was pregnant and that Dad's invention allowed not only me, but many other diabetic women to be able to safely carry a baby to full term, with the ability to monitor their sugar levels at home.

Most of the patients, at this stage, would come to me with their Medicare cards so I would not have to leave my seat. I thought this was such a considerate deed from all of them however, I was still willing and extremely able to move myself around quite comfortably. I always had a zest in my step so although their best thoughts were there, I used to say to them that I was able to and wanting to get up and have a stretch.

After the last patient left on this one quiet afternoon I approached the doctor, our normal daily routine was to speak about the day and make sure everything was finalised prior to us leaving the surgery. He did not look his normal relaxed self at the end of this particular day. This was quite unusual as we would always go down to the kitchen and have a coffee or a tea and discuss the day's events, together with any planning requirements for the following day. I made a coffee for both of us, which was the normal routine and sat down after a what was, so far, turning out to be a different day in so many ways. Firstly, the pathology call, then the unusually quiet and early end of the day. For me, everything just seemed different, and I was feeling slightly uneasy for some strange reason. I was just about to receive some terrible news…

Once we were sitting down at the table which was positioned in the sunlight, I was informed by the doctor that the pathology contacted him about my pregnancy blood test results. I asked if everything was OK and as having diabetes for 20 years, I was concerned that I would get some news that my diabetes was giving me some trouble. I was slightly confused as my sugar levels were constantly monitored, thanks to my Dad's invention, and I rarely had any test results throughout any time of the day that were not within the normal range. I would monitor constantly throughout each day to make sure my glucose control was perfectly balanced. I had always, prior to being pregnant, had extremely tight control so I was adamant that my sugar levels during my pregnancy would be very tightly monitored to prevent any damage being caused to my unborn baby.

I was told by the doctor that my diabetes had absolutely nothing to do with my test results and I was then informed that I had Rhesus Antibodies showing in my blood. I was absolutely unaware of what this meant, and it was very well explained to me by the doctor that I had worked with for many years. Although I was in absolute shock and fear, I was extremely comforted that I had the support of someone I knew very well who was able to explain what the concern was and what the next step would be. As I was 32 weeks pregnant at this stage, I was extremely fearful that I could, at this late stage of a perfect pregnancy, lose my baby.

I was told that somehow my negative blood type had crossed over to my baby's positive blood type and as we had different blood groups, this basically meant that my blood was now identifying my baby as a foreign object. My body was therefore creating antibodies to fight the crossover of my baby's blood. This was extremely worrying and after a call to my husband, at the time, my pregnancy was in jeopardy and there was a chance that I could lose my baby.

We immediately made our way to my Obstetrician in Sydney as the doctor I worked for was the one that contacted the Obstetrician to inform him of my condition. It was at this stage, I understood this was the outside line he had asked for earlier that day.

On arrival to the specialist's surgery, which was located directly across the road from the hospital, I was taken in immediately. It was explained to me exactly what was happening, and it was made clear that further tests were required to ascertain the nature of the damage done to my baby by the antibodies. I was sent to a hospital near Hornsby, as this was where the specialist was located, and this would be where the amniocentesis was to be performed. We lived on the Central Coast of NSW which was located about half an hour north of Hornsby, so it was good that it was on our way home anyway.

It was explained to me that a long needle would be placed into my tummy and into the amniotic fluid of which a sample would be taken. The amniotic fluid would give the specialist an accurate level of the antibodies which were destroying my baby. It was a very unpleasant experience and at 32 weeks pregnant, there was a high risk of me going into early labour.

After a couple of hours of being monitored following the amniocentesis, the results had come back from the pathology lab. I was told that the antibody levels were safe enough to leave my baby in the womb for further development. I was sent home and was told I would be extremely tightly monitored for further increases in my antibody levels. My levels of antibodies could now be monitored via a blood test, so this was carried out weekly.

At 35 weeks pregnant, it was decided by my Obstetrician and the specialist who carried out the amniocentesis that my baby would be born by caesarean section at 36 weeks. This would mean that the baby would be large enough to survive after birth due to the pregnancy time, although there was a real concern that my baby would be extremely sick when born and would require an intense amount of medical intervention post birth.

I was admitted to hospital on 30th July 1992. I arrived at approximately midday and was taken to a room within the maternity section of the hospital. The maternity section was a building on its own and was incorporated with a birthing suite, an operating theatre, as well as a neo natal intensive care ward. The neo natal intensive care ward was upstairs with the operating theatre and birthing suites, on the lower level were the private and public patient rooms. Half of the rooms had been renovated and I was lucky enough to have one of the newly renovated, very modern, and comfortable rooms.

I was nervous about the following day as it would be the day my baby was going to be born. The theatre was booked for 9am so I was woken incredibly early in the morning for a shower and preparation for my caesarean section. My concern was mainly due to the possible unwell nature of my baby and although the weight was good for a 36-week baby, it was the rhesus antibodies and their concerning interaction that was at the forefront of my mind. The delivery did not come soon enough for me. As I am a nervous patient, I chose to be put under a general anaesthetic for the surgery. I also did not want my stress to affect my baby during the caesarean section.

CHAPTER 26

# MY FIRST BORN

At 9.51am on 31$^{st}$ July 1992, I gave birth to a beautiful but very unwell baby boy. He was 6lb 3oz and was immediately rushed to the neonatal intensive care unit for further testing and immediate treatment. I was in the recovery ward for several days, they were concerned that I had not been able to see my baby, due to his intensive care requirements. I was also in a tremendous amount of pain, so they kept me in the recovery suite for a longer time than normal. When the time came for me to be able to visit my baby boy, Mitchell, I would be close enough to visit when I could.

The first time I saw him, I was wheeled to see him through a window which was purposely set up for any new mother who could not gain direct access to their newborn baby. It was the hardest emotion I had ever had to experience not being able to pick my baby up and hold him in my arms. I was expressing breast milk, so he was fed with my milk through a tube. It was day three after his birth that I was able to lay eyes on my new baby boy.

After going through such emotional turmoil with his sickness, this, mixed with tears of joy as I stared in awe at my beautiful baby boy watching him breathe and lay in his humidicrib so helpless. They finally took me to my own private hospital room downstairs. At this stage I was determined to return to the neonatal intensive care ward to see my baby repeatedly. After approximately five days, I was going to visit him using the elevator and I would now be able to enter the intensive care ward and, after several intensive hand washing procedures, I was able to hold his little hand and stroke his head. This was the most incredible and emotional experience that at my young age of twenty-five had ever encountered.

Poor little Mitch required three blood transfusions to stop the antibodies destroying his blood. His bilirubin levels were completely out of their normal range, and he only had a twenty percent chance of survival due to the antibodies. This was absolutely and totally heartbreaking for me as my baby boy was subjected to a mother with diabetes, which entailed an enormous amount of risk during a pregnancy. Thankfully, the only risk was me not controlling my sugar levels and thankfully with my Dad's brilliant invention, I had great control with my glucose levels, I was now thankfully the proud Mum of a baby that was not affected in any way by bad control.

I stayed in hospital for a week after having Mitchell. He was struggling but he had good fight in him which thankfully enabled him to take small steps forward every day. He was not out of the woods yet as he was premature and still very unwell and sadly, I was sent home without him. This was an emotional experience which I would not wish upon anyone, and I certainly had not given the thought of going home without my baby any consideration.

I returned daily to the neonatal intensive care unit and spent about eight hours a day sitting beside the humidicrib watching my baby boy take each breath and hoping that the miraculous work from the committed staff would be enough to make my baby healthy enough to take home. This was difficult to comprehend as he was covered in tubes, which therefore made it impossible to have a cuddle. I desperately wanted to hold my little Mitch and although the staff felt it was important for me to bond physically with my baby, I did not want to jeopardise his recovery so therefore just sat beside him and held his little hand through the humidicrib.

As the days passed, Mitch was starting to improve and his colour was becoming a normal baby colour, not a jaundice yellow baby which was caused by the bilirubin levels in his blood. Thankfully, the antibodies were reducing as the blood transfusions were starting to take effect. It was at this stage that I began to feel confident that my baby was going to be OK.

Mitch was able to leave the neonatal intensive care unit when he was four weeks old. His weight was increasing rapidly as I had been expressing milk during my time at home and I would visit the hospital and take my milk in an esky to the neonatal ward. The staff would store my breast milk and feed Mitchell through a tube every two hours. I did spend an intense week, prior to the hospital allowing him to go home with me, training how to breast feed my baby. As he was unable to be breast fed immediately after birth, it was a slow and important process that required expert and very patient help from the hospital staff.

My most emotional day as a young Mum was felt with elation and happiness but also the emotions were with intense trepidation and fear of taking a still not so well or strong baby home from hospital. I had never been a Mum before and really did not know how to look after a new baby, other than what the neonatal intensive care unit nurses had taught me. It was not like an average "new Mum" experience as Mitchell was now four weeks old and I had never had him sleep in the same room as me overnight. The mother's care of a newborn baby is something that a full-term birth without any complications starts immediately. This is something that I did not have the opportunity to experience.

It now made sense to me why my Mum would show me unconditional love and care to help me with anything I needed. I knew that my own Mum would be there for absolutely anything. Mum and Dad were over the moon with their first grandchild being a little boy, my Dad would have loved having his own son and with me being their only child, along with being a girl. My Dad would have loved his own little boy... He certainly loved me and taught me some incredible things that a girl usually would not be interested in. My Dad had an amazing ability to make anything he put his mind to look easy and fun. This is why I loved spending time with my Dad in his workshop. I considered myself absolutely blessed that he taught me some wonderful and incredible skills such as soldering, working with electronics, making model cars and planes together with an array of simple car repairs and how technical gadgets worked. I was certain that Dad would thoroughly enjoy his new Grandson by teaching him all the things he taught me.

## CHAPTER 27

# NEW DEVELOPMENT

As our blood glucose monitor business had virtually ended and Dad was now carrying out any repairs to his glucose testers at home, it was imperative for him to earn an income. He was interested in a property development opportunity which basically came about from a person both Mum and Dad knew. There was the possibility of purchasing a caravan park in Tuncurry and with the help of quite a few investors, the caravan park would become a villa park. Both Mum and Dad agreed to become part of this new venture and therefore put a large chunk of their savings into the project. It was a perfect block of land for a significant number of villas and after having plans drawn up, the council very quickly gave approval for the project to begin.

This was overly exciting as Dad now had a new income opportunity to look forward to and as the project was originally planned to take approximately nine months to complete, Mum and Dad took comfort in knowing that they would now have enough money coming through the door. With Mum's job at the doctor's surgery, as well as their remaining savings, they would manage financially until the building project was completed. My Mum had taken over my job at the doctor's surgery when I left to have Mitch, Mum's job was three or four days a week so both Mum and Dad knew they could secure their income for future years.

Within a month of the approval being granted by the council, the land was cleared, and the tractors moved in to level the site and begin preparation for construction to commence. Progress was extremely fast and thankfully the weather played an important role in the continuous flow of the project. Mum and Dad made a few trips from their home to Tuncurry on the mid north coast of NSW to visit the building site and inspect the progress of the villa complex. They were extremely impressed with its development, and they felt they had made the right decision to enter into this new joint venture with five other investors who also believed the project would be a lucrative one. It seemed the builder knew what he was doing, and the project management of the complex was very well controlled. There were no problems with delivery of wood, windows, plumbing or electrical items and the progress was fast and perfectly accurate.

Within a few months, the project came to a halt. The complex required more products and finances before it could be finalised, and this was something that the partners could not afford. Due to the building progress being put on standby for months, some of the partners almost lost their homes as they had mortgaged them to fund the project.

Thankfully, Mum and Dad were recommended to a powerful solicitor in Sydney and together with their own accountant they were able to walk away from the experience with minimal loss. The whole ordeal was extremely stressful for the two of them, and it was a cruel blow after losing such a successful business with the glucose testers.

CHAPTER 28

# CARD READING

During the time of the Tuncurry villa development project, Dad bought a book of vouchers from a local charity. It was a fund-raising booklet whereby local businesses donated their time and products for the fund-raising company to make money for charity. One of the vouchers was for a tarot card reading at Narrabeen. I had been going through a horrid time with my husband recently leaving Mitchell and myself, so I decided to contact the tarot card reader to book an appointment. I felt that nothing more could go wrong for me at that time so therefore felt comfortable that any news I would be given from the tarot card reader would be a breath of fresh air compared to the last 6 to 12 months I had endured. With my marriage break up, together with my Mum and Dad going through a few torturous years, Murphy's Law prevailed and what could go wrong, did go wrong. I thought it would be a good idea to take advantage of having my cards read. I booked the appointment for the following afternoon and decided to ask Dad to drop me to the shop which was next to the main bus station at Narrabeen which overlooked the lake. The lake always had an abundance of windsurfers, canoes and fishing boats and it was always a beautiful location to visit and relax.

On arrival, I was jewellery free and car key free, and this was a deliberate decision on my part as I did not want to offer any hints to the card reader about my life. As this was the first card reading I had ever experienced, I was extremely sceptical so therefore limited any information as to where I lived etc. I simply introduced myself as Lisa and sat where the card reading would take place. I was asked to shuffle the cards, which was a slight joke as I certainly could not shuffle cards without dropping them all over the place. Thankfully, when I shuffled the cards, I did not drop one. I was then asked to select a few cards and lay them on the table in front of me. Once I had laid them out on the table, the tarot reader said, "you poor thing, you have been through hell lately". I was gobsmacked as this person that I had never met before and had absolutely no information about my life, was able to tell that I had been through a rough time.

She then asked me to select a few more cards out of the pile and lay them in different locations on the table. I was then informed that I was going to meet someone that had a large involvement with paper. I honestly thought that I had made an appointment with a fruit loop person as that was quite a specific prediction and as I had never had my cards read before, I was unaware how the process worked. I certainly did not know that extremely specific details could be brought about on a tarot card. My head was spinning, wondering what the paper meant. Funnily enough, my first thought was toilet paper and then, for months after my reading, I forgot the paper comment and moved on with my life and did not give the subject any further thought.

CHAPTER 29

# PAPER MEETING

At the time of the development project failure, I was introduced to a man who was a sales representative for the local newspaper. Amazingly, the tarot card reader had predicted this meeting and I was bewildered as to how she knew the man I was to meet would be heavily involved in paper. He too had lost his wife to her having an affair, so our stories were terribly similar. We both had friends who lived across the road from each other, and it was our friends that decided they would set up a dinner for six of us to get together and hopefully create a friendship between myself and the paper man.

I saw it as a blind date, and this was something that I certainly was not really interested in although I was grateful to my friends for thinking of me and arranging a dinner for me. It would be a dinner for them, their neighbours, myself, and a man I had never met so I approached the idea with the greatest of trepidation, however I felt obliged to agree to it as they had been fabulous friends both before but more so after Mitchell's Dad had left us. They had twin boys the same age as Mitchell, so Mitch and I spent many days with the twins and their Mum going to the park, playing in the backyard as we drank coffee and watched them.

After reluctantly agreeing to a blind date, it was established that the three of us girls would create the meal for six people. My friend created entrée, her neighbour created a main meal, and I was left to create dessert. I decided to make a trifle which was a light yet extremely tasty dessert and, as always, I made it sugar free. It was my Mum's recipe which she had made ever since I was a little girl. It was always such a success that I felt obligated to do my beautiful Mum justice and use her recipe.

I was going to stay at my friend's house that night, so I would not have to wake my 18-month-old toddler from his sleep to take him home. He was being looked after by my friend's eldest child and as I was only across the road, I was confident that Mitchell was in good and safe hands. After all, she had twin bothers the same age as Mitchell. I was thankful for the night off being a Mum and could enjoy myself which, as a single Mum, was something that did not happen often.

Although neither of us two blind date candidates did not fall head over heels with each other at first sight, we were both polite for the sake of our friends and did, however, have a fun night. I made a big impression with my Mum's amazing trifle recipe and the night was a success for all of us with great laughter and good stories to share. The following morning, there was a knock at my friend's front door. It was the paper man, Craig, my blind date from the previous night's dinner. He had stayed at his friend's home for the night also and his friends told him that morning that he needed to go across the road and ask Lisa out for a coffee. He was given no choice about the matter.

My friend answered the door and Craig asked if I was there. As I had heard his voice, I walked out of the kitchen and was asked by Craig if I wanted to go out with him for a coffee. My friend was more than happy to look after Mitchell for a few hours, so we ventured to nearby Terrigal beach and our very first date consisted of a walk along the promenade before grabbing a coffee at one of the many coffee shops. Neither of us were short on conversation however our main discussion was how the two of us were extremely upset that our previous cheating partners had taken advantage of the trust that both Craig and I felt was a very important part in a marriage. We discussed this, amongst other topics, and after a few great hours of light-hearted conversation we returned to our friends' homes to thank them for arranging a lovely night, we then both went back to our respective homes.

Neither of us felt any real spark for each other, although we did enjoy being able to discuss many topics, we also enjoyed each other's company, conversation, and laughter.

The following day, I received a call from Craig asking if he could come to my house for dinner. I felt sorry for him as he had mentioned to me that he was living on 2-minute microwave cheeseburgers and 2-minute noodles. I thought it was about time he had some vegetables and a good hearty meal. I was concerned that he was wanting to visit me, not only to get a good meal but I was also thinking he may have been expecting something that I wasn't prepared to "offer" on a second meeting. Thankfully, the subject did not come up during our conversation and after a quick peck on the cheek, Craig left having showed the utmost respect for me.

He contacted me a couple of days later and asked if he could come for dinner a second time. As we enjoyed our conversations, I once again agreed. At the end of the night, after another quick peck on the cheek, Craig left. The next time he called me, he asked me to visit him, and he would take me out for dinner to a Thai restaurant located at The Entrance. During our dinner, Craig decided to show off and ate a whole chilli. Neither of us had much previous experience eating chilli so it was an unknown as to what effect this would have on him. Within a few seconds of eating the chilli, Craig became extremely agitated and went completely red in his eyes and his face. He had perspiration dripping down his face and he could barely talk. Although I was concerned, I could not stop laughing at him for even attempting to eat an entire chilli in one mouthful. After several glasses of milk, which the restaurant staff provided, I realised it was not a laughing matter, this was serious, a few minutes later Craig was able to speak again and had cooled down.

We laughed all night and he said all he wanted to do was impress me. He not only impressed me, but he made me laugh like I had not laughed since my marriage break up 12 months prior. It was at this stage, we both realised we liked each other, and a good friendship had begun.

As the weeks progressed and our friendship grew, Craig had a previously booked holiday to visit his family on Norfolk Island. His holiday was booked for three weeks and as we had just met, the lovesick Craig was ringing me from a Norfolk Island phone box nearly every day. He laughingly mentioned that he was feeding the phone box with coins every thirty seconds. The calls were becoming very expensive when he decided that writing letters was a cheaper option. The love letters he wrote me were beautiful and we still have them to this day.

We were both very comfortable with each other's company and decided we were going to stay together as boyfriend and girlfriend. After about a year of our blind date dinner, Craig was offered a promotion with his job in the newspapers. The position meant that he would need to travel for an hour each way up and down the freeway. As our relationship was strong and we wanted to be together on a more permanent basis, Craig moved in with Mitchell and I as my home at the time was only half an hour travel to his new office. Craig was enjoying his new position and our relationship was going strong. Our new family of three was becoming solid, Craig and I knew that we were in love and could not be without each other. Definitely a lot to be said for my tarot card reading, she was certainly right with her prediction!

CHAPTER 30

# PREPARE FOR TAKEOFF

It was shortly after this time, in 1994, that my Dad had the opportunity to purchase a small airplane. He had always wanted to learn to fly so he thought it would be a good idea to purchase the plane and use it to have his learner lessons in. He met a man who had an instructor's licence, and he was more than happy to go with Dad to inspect the plane and take it out flying for a short period of time to make sure it was of sound condition and suitable to learn to fly in. The plane passed with flying colours and Dad was happy with his small investment. It was a 2-seater plane but certainly was not a Learjet or jumbo jet. Its structure was impeccable and although it was not the most comfortable ride, it was perfect for Dad to learn to fly.

Dad had spent several lessons with his instructor learning in a larger plane at Bankstown Airport. Thankfully, Dad loved his flying and was very happy that he had purchased his own plane. Although he was not yet able to fly solo, he found a hanger not far from my home on the Central Coast of NSW. It was a short 5-minute drive from my home and was lucky to have a very private runway which rarely saw any aircraft take off or land. It was very affordable accommodation for my Dad's aircraft, so Dad was more than confident with his aircraft's new home. He knew it would be looked after and he also knew that when he had his own licence, he could conveniently drop Mum off to my place, which was a one-hour drive away from their home and then a further five minutes from my place to the airport.

As Dad continued his lessons down in Sydney, his new purchase was flown by the old owner to the hanger. This was a very exciting day for Dad as he had always wanted to fly. It was an absolute thrill not only for Dad, but also Mum and I, that he could look forward to doing something he loved. A note to the reader, It is not normally in my nature to hold a grudge and I can generally let things slide in my life however, what happened to Dad was heartbreaking for me. Dad had suffered a major blow losing his successful company through no fault of his own. It was the multinational companies that made Dad feel worthless by taking something away from him that he had successfully built from his pure love for me. My Dad felt he had failed, which to this day is something that still breaks my heart. I would always say to Dad that absolutely no one could take away from him, or from our small family of three, what he had created. A truly remarkable invention which became a major phenomenon in the lives of every type 1 and type 2 diabetics as well as their family members and friends.

Several months later, Dad's plane required its yearly registration check. As Dad was not yet endorsed to fly his plane, he asked if his instructor would fly his plane, along with Dad, to Cessnock airport where the plane needed to go for its check. His instructor was honoured that he had asked him and agreed immediately. He became good friends with Dad during the lessons and Dad was aware that he and his wife had been trying for a baby for quite some time. When he agreed to fly Dad and his plane to Cessnock, Dad thought that it would be a good day out for his instructor, and it might help his frame of mind.

At this time, I was doing a computer course at Gosford technical college, so my Mum would come to my place to look after Mitchell. He was about 18 months old at the time and Mitchell's Dad had left us both when Mitchell was only six months old. My Mum and Dad were spending plenty of time with Mitchell and myself and were my support through not only daily life but my many challenges of being a young Mum with a young child. Mitchell absolutely cherished every moment he spent with my Mum and Dad and would look forward to any opportunity to see his Nanna and Grandad. Although he was young, when I mentioned Nanna and Grandad, Mitch would get a priceless grin on his cute little face and would say "Nanna and ga-ga". Mitch could not say Grandad, so he used to call my Dad "ga-ga". So cute...

It was bright and early one beautiful sunny and balmy day where Mum and Dad made the drive from the northern beaches, up the F3, which later changed its name to the M1. They were on their way to come to my home and later Dad was to meet the instructor at the airport where Dad kept his plane. It was registration test day for Dad's new pride and joy, it was the first time that the plane was to be used under Dad's ownership. I left to attend my training course and as was my normal routine, I left Mitchell with Mum. She was going to stay at my place with Mitchell for the day while Dad was going to meet his instructor at the airport.

The weather was fabulous. Mitchell wanted to go with his Grandad to see his new plane so Mum decided to take Mitchell and drive with Dad to the airport. Mum thought that it would be a perfect opportunity to see Dad fulfill his dream of being in his own plane and together with Mitchell having the excitement of seeing his Grandad fly off down the runway, it would also give Mitchell the thrill of seeing an airplane close-up and be able to climb inside it and check out what the inside of a cockpit looked like. Mitch had a very strong interest for anything to do with airplanes, so Mum was excited to see the reaction of both Dad and Mitch doing something together that they were both so passionate about.

After the plane's preparation for the flight and finding Mum and Mitch a suitable viewing point for the plane's take-off, Dad and his instructor carried out the required pre-flight checks. Following all the steps necessary for a safe flight. Together, they strapped on their seatbelts making perfectly sure there were no safety or mechanical issues they had possibly missed. They had also been keeping an eye, during the previous few days, on the weather. Everything was in check, and they were ready for take-off for the half hour flight. Dad had filled the petrol tank and it was always his concern that he would run out of petrol. This was something we used to joke around about, but it was a fear that he always had so he was adamant that he would ensure the fuel tank was full to the brim.

As they taxied to the end of the runway, they once again did all the necessary checks to ensure they would have a trouble free and enjoyable flight. Dad's heart was racing as this experience was something he deserved after a previous horrible few years of nothing but disappointment. My Dad never felt sorry for himself, it was simply the fact that he felt he had failed other people so to finally achieve his lifetime ambition and be able to fly was something that really did put a smile on his face.

They received clearance to take off and they were watched by a very excited Mitch and Mum. What a perfect day for Dad's first flight in his new toy. They were absolutely blessed with picture perfect weather and virtually no wind at all. The plane left the runway and after a fabulous, non-eventful take off, it was a time for celebration. Dad was one hundred percent confident that his little plane was perfect in every way, and he had made the right decision to purchase it.

Mum had spoken with Dad about insurance for the plane and as he felt that the airport it was kept at was well secured, he did not feel the need to insure it. He said to Mum that if he crashes the plane, he will probably die anyway and then Mum would get his life insurance, so she would not have any financial worries. It was also something that we would talk and laugh about, we all agreed that people rarely survive a plane crash. After many discussions about insurance of the plane, both Mum and Dad decided that insurance was a cost that was not necessary.

As Mitch had that priceless excited grin on his face, it seemed the take-off was perfect and quick as a flash, Mum and Mitch watched the plane drop below the tree line as it made an almighty crash to the ground. The airport was in a bush setting and the area surrounding the airstrip was dense bushland. Mum drew a sharp breath not believing what she just saw and the sound of the plane hitting trees and crashing to the ground with a grinding thud, thankfully Mitch, being so young, did not understand quite what was happening.

The airport was isolated, and the area was mostly farms and bush land, so the local properties were spread far and wide which is why my poor Mum went into a state of panic and immense concern as to where my Dad's plane went down. Mobile phones were only just becoming a new technology, so she frustratingly had no way of contacting the authorities and rescue teams to jump into action and find Dad, his pilot, and the plane crash site. She also contemplated with dread the idea that my Dad, the man that had successfully aided so many people around the world with his invention, could very possibly be lying dead or seriously injured in a paddock or bushland somewhere. With Mum being panic stricken and together with making sure her 18-month-old grandson was safe and in a comfortable environment, my poor Mum was promptly forced to make a very difficult decision. As she did not know the area, other than the airport, she needed to decide where to go and which direction to take. As the airport was so small, there were rarely any people around so she could not gain the assistance from anyone.

She put Mitchell in his car seat, shaking with fear and concern, and decided to head back to my house as she knew that direction and knew that it would only be a quick five-minute drive to be able to use my home phone to contact the necessary authorities. Thankfully, close to the entrance of the airport, she noticed a large double story house which looked very quiet. She was concerned that if she went to the house, and left the airport, she would be wasting time if no one was home. The house had a three-car garage however there were no cars in the driveway, Mum was hoping and praying that someone would be there to answer when she knocked on the door.

Mum parked the car in the driveway of the house. Still shaking and fearful, she raced up the front staircase to the front door. It seems the elderly gentleman that lived there had noticed Mum drive her car onto his property so before she had a chance to knock on the door, the gentleman opened the door and immediately noticed her alarmed state. My Mum was normally a very mentally strong person and could deal with whatever challenges life presented however this was a different and stressful scenario.

She knew that this could be a potential tragedy. A million thoughts were going through her head, and it was at this stage, having found someone who had a clear line of thinking that could make the necessary calls. She could now concentrate on Mitch to ensure he did not notice the emotional turmoil that was going on around him. In a very hurried and with a slightly rambling voice, she explained to the owner of the house what had just happened.

The elderly gentleman immediately made a phone call to "000" and informed them of the dire situation. The airport runway could be seen from his front balcony however the occupant of the home was not at this location when the accident happened so therefore did not witness the plane going down.

The police, ambulance, fire, and rescue where there within about 10 minutes, together with the local newspaper. They were not sure exactly where the plane had gone down so it was extremely important that Mum gave them a clear description of the altitude and location as closely as she could. This was hard for Mum because although she knew that the authorities were there to help, seeing them arrive so very close together meant that her concern about losing my Dad may very soon be realised.

The reality of this was very emotionally painful for her as this also meant that her future may very well be changed forever in the blink of an eye. As the paramedics rallied around her and Mitch, their immediate priority was to make sure that both Mum and Mitch were emotionally OK after the turmoil of them both witnessing what had just happened. While they were being monitored, the other members of the relevant emergency services made the dash to find the plane. This was not an easy task as although they knew the plane had gone down reasonably close to the airport, the bushland and freeway which was surrounding the airport, was quite dense. They did not know what they were about to be faced with and what may be the worst outcome for all involved.

Once Mum and Mitch were assessed by the paramedics, they were both given the all-clear and were then consulted by the investigating police officers informing Mum that the crash site was located in bushland very close to the freeway. The plane had flipped over and landed on the ground upside down, large tree branches strewn everywhere, the engine and propeller of the plane had sheared off and landed in a nearby dam. It was not clear at this stage if my Dad or his instructor had survived. Mum desperately needed to know the exact condition of the pilot and, more importantly, Dad. However, what was made very clear to Mum was that the plane wasn't in a very good way. It was going to be quite a task to muster the necessary equipment to retrieve the crashed aircraft.

Thankfully, the team worked extremely hard and fast and were able to access the crash site in a reasonably short period of time. As they had been set the task of going through dense bushland, their line of sight prior to arriving at the scene was very limited so they were therefore quite concerned what they might be confronted with. After all, the plane had landed on its roof, so the cabin had been somewhat crushed and buried in a pile of dirt. Arriving at the crash site, they found a dazed and confused man standing near the aircraft. They did not know how many occupants were on the plane at the time of the crash and needed to investigate that situation immediately, however knowing there was at least one conscious survivor was hopeful relief. He was somewhat still very capable and was presenting with remarkable cognitive thought and the rescue squad were informed by the surviving occupant that he had kicked his way out of the cabin. This was a mammoth task for the survivor as the windscreen and cabin was made from a very strong Perspex and timber construction.

It was then, within a short time after discovering the surviving occupant standing beside the plane that they discovered that there was only one other occupant, the pilot, who was trapped upside down inside the cabin and was sadly unable to communicate. At this stage, they did not know if the trapped pilot had survived the plane crash so the rescue squad got the paramedics to assess him so they could then ensure the next necessary steps they could take to remove the trapped patient from the crashed plane. This was going to be difficult as the location of the wreckage was in an area that not only had very difficult access but was made additionally challenging with most of the crash site being surrounded with barbed wire fencing. This was something that would certainly hinder a very prompt recovery of the trapped pilot as they required a large amount of specialised equipment to remove him safely from the plane.

After the paramedics assessed the patient, they informed the surviving occupant that the trapped person was still alive but was unconscious. They were not able to properly assess him until he could be released from the wreckage, and they also knew that this could take some time as the patient's safe removal was of paramount importance. Thankfully, his vital signs were strong, and they administered a saline drip until the rescue team were able to extract him from the wreckage. It was unclear at this stage whether he had any broken bones or was trapped by his legs or arms. It was going to be a slow process and although the patient was alive, it still was not a great scenario for him to be trapped in an upside-down plane for a great length of time.

The rescue people were extraordinarily quick to cut through the barbed wire fencing and gradually remove the damaged cockpit of the plane. It was also very important that removing any part of the plane could impact heavily on the state and safety of the occupant, so it was important to be executed in a precise and expert manner. The team worked tirelessly for about an hour before they were able to remove the patient safely and as painlessly for him as possible. He was still unconscious however after the intense work from the paramedics and with the excellent teamwork from all the authorities involved, the occupant was alive and did not have any broken bones or major cuts. His entire body was covered in mild lacerations however they were mainly concerned about his unconscious state.

At this point, I was still unaware of my Dad's plane crash. I was at my computer course so had not been informed about the situation as my Mum did not want to concern me or spoil my opportunity for me to learn something that I really wanted to fulfill.

Mum was informed by the authorities that both the occupants had survived the crash although she was not given any further details, she was instructed to meet the ambulances down at the hospital. Thankfully, the gentleman that helped Mum during the experience offered to drive both her and Mitchell to the hospital as he was concerned that she wasn't in a safe enough frame of mind to drive her own car. Mum waited with Mitchell as the gentleman locked his home and then unlocked his garage downstairs. On opening the garage door, my Mum noticed a stunning Silver Shadow Rolls Royce in the garage, and she thought it was a collectable car that he used on special occasions only. Within a minute or two, the car was waiting for Mum to put Mitchell's car seat in, Mum was totally overwhelmed that as Dad was being transported by ambulance to the hospital, Mum and Mitchell were being driven in one very expensive and beautifully appointed form of transport. The hospital was approximately 15 minutes away from the airport, so she had very worrying thoughts not knowing what state my Dad was in, or the instructor for that matter, together with the conflicting thoughts of being driven to the hospital in such a luxurious car.

Mum arrived at the hospital before the ambulances as the paramedics had to be careful to make sure the patient did not have any back or neck injuries. They drove very slowly to ensure they did not cause any further damage. Mum was unable to enter the emergency department, so she had to sit in the waiting room with Mitchell and it was at this point that Mum found a moment to contact me at the college and inform me of what had happened. With my despair and shock at the news she had just given me, I immediately packed up my things and made the incredibly anxious trip to the hospital.

Shortly after making the call to me, she was taken through to the emergency department and informed about the condition of both surviving plane crash victims. It was news that she certainly needed to hear as she was told that Dad, other than a few scratches, was in perfect condition and would be able to leave the hospital after a couple of hours of observation. Sadly, the instructor was not in as good a condition as Dad. He had thankfully regained consciousness and was given the clearance of a broken back, neck, or any other bone fractures. Both Mum and Dad were extremely relieved that his wife would be told that her husband had survived a plane crash. He still had injuries, which were severe bruising and lacerations to several parts of his body and due to this, he was required to stay in hospital for observation for a week following the plane crash. Both men were very lucky to survive such a catastrophic incident.

As Dad left the emergency department, one of the nurses suggested to him that he should purchase a lottery ticket. Although he had a quick thought that buying a lottery ticket was not a bad idea, he responded by saying he believed he had used all his luck up by surviving a plane crash. It is certainly something that not very many people can truthfully say they have lived through such an incredible event. This was an extremely relieving time for my Mum as she knew that she did not need to contemplate life without my Dad and she was thankful that the outcome was somewhat of a happy ending, rather than a terrible result. After all, it was only the loss of an aircraft and not the loss of her husband's life.

It was shortly after Dad's release from hospital that he was required to carry out an in-depth interview of the process and the events leading up to and also including the time of the accident. This was a difficult time for Dad as it forced him to relive what he had just been through so this was a very emotionally stressful event yet at the same time, Dad was fully aware that he had literally just survived a plane crash. Very mixed emotions emerged during the interview. Dad's information of exactly what happened lead the authorities to believe that the cause of the accident was by mother nature in the form of wind shear. After further investigations, it was confirmed that Dad's plane crashed by something that neither Dad or his instructor friend had any cause or control over. Apparently, what happened was as the aircraft was gaining altitude, after the end of the runway, wind shear had pushed the aircraft down onto the top of the tree canopy which promptly stopped the plane in its tracks and flipped it over and it then crashed to the ground upside down. This news was a major relief for both Mum and Dad and although Dad's plane was beyond repair and was not covered by any insurance, both Dad and the pilot were not guilty of any wrongdoing.

Thankfully, Dad's instructor friend was released from hospital after the week of being monitored and with an absolute miraculous turn of events, within three months of the plane crash, he and his wife were welcomed with the fabulous news they were expecting a baby. They welcomed their healthy baby nine months later and although Mum and Dad stayed connected with them for many years after the crash, sadly they did lose contact with each other over time.

# CHAPTER 31

# LAST VOCATION

As Dad spent months recovering from the emotional and physical turmoil of his accident, he used his time to clean out his many workshops around the house where he stored all his tools and remaining equipment from the factory. Keeping in mind, that if he kept himself busy, he would forget what had happened and he could move forward. The remains of the plane were sold to a fellow plane enthusiast who would use the parts and modify them for the building of another plane. This certainly did help and within about six months after the accident Dad was thankfully able to laugh about what had happened, simply saying that he had never met anyone in his life that had miraculously survived a plane crash. He bought the odd lottery ticket at this stage however sadly none of them were winners. He did say that if he did win the lottery, he certainly would not use the winnings to buy another plane.

Dad had been contemplating for many months what he wanted to do with his remaining years of work. He had sadly lost the opportunity of becoming financially successful with the Tuncurry building project so he knew that he would have to find a job to keep the money coming through the front door. Mums job at the doctor's surgery continued for quite some time, however as it was only a few days a week, there was not enough money to stay afloat with their bills. Dad was in constant contact with his friends and was approached by Bob, his long-term friend that he worked with at Hanimex many years before. Bob mentioned to Dad that he was working for a company that produced sleep apnoea equipment. Bob said that they required a research and development expert to join their small team of employees. Dad was extremely excited at the possibility of working with Bob again as they had a fabulous working relationship. After all, working well together is what originally started their friendship. An appointment was set up with the CEO of the company and my Dad was offered a job immediately. The company was at Macquarie Park in the Ryde area of Sydney so the travel every day for Dad was not of any concern, as it was a reasonably easy and straight forward trip.

Dad had worked for himself for many years so to work for someone else who could possibly dictate to him what his every working hour would entail was something Dad was slightly apprehensive about. His first week was a major learning curve although my Dad always loved to discover new technology and techniques, so he really enjoyed his new job. Dad's boss knew of his background and was also aware that Dad had created the world's first home glucose tester, so he was confident that Dad was extremely self-motivated and capable of virtually anything.

He very quickly, after Dad's training time, allowed him to work alone without being supervised around the clock. He also knew that Dad was able to create new products based on research. Dad settled into the company extremely quickly and it was only a matter of time before my Dad, using his capable knowledge and inventive nature, developed a miniature sleep apnoea breathing mask that would better fit babies and children. This was a very important project as all available masks only fitted adults so the use of a sleep apnoea machine for babies and children was difficult yet extremely necessary.

As Dads work continued and the company he worked for was rapidly growing, he was also aware that Mum was no longer happy at the doctor's surgery and wanted to find another job. The timing was perfect as Dad was informed that the company which he was working for required someone to enter their team in the accounts department. This was Mums forte and within a short time, Mum had a job interview with the CEO. This was the same person that gave Dad his start with the company. Mum was then employed in their accounts department and for many years, Mum and Dad would make the trip to and from work every day in the same car. This was a financial bonus and now that Mum was not travelling to the surgery for work, they were able to save money on petrol.

ResMed was becoming an extremely large company and within the time Mum and Dad worked for them, they moved twice to larger premises and continued growing. The initial employees became very good friends and as the company grew, they were placed in different parts of the new building. They all had varying roles, so the different departments became further apart as the company grew into its new premises. The initial building where Dad was first employed was a small office block and the parking was extremely limited. There was certainly enough space and parking for the employees at ResMed however ResMed's next two buildings consisted of massive office spaces. They had much larger parking areas along with workshop and lab type facilities within. The latter buildings were built with a level of luxury that certainly did not exist in the first building.

## CHAPTER 32

# THE PROPOSAL

By this stage, my Mum and Dad were the happiest they had been for several years, and the planets seemed to really be aligning for them. Although they were like any normal couple with their ups and downs, they had found comfort in knowing that they were both lucky enough to have great jobs with great colleagues that they thoroughly enjoyed. This was a blessing for the two of them as they had been through years of disappointment and loss. Craig and I were also in a fabulous place in our lives. Craig got down on one knee and proposed to me one evening as I was washing up after dinner. I thought he was joking so I laughed at him, continued to wash the dishes, and replied with a very strong "NO". Sadly, I did upset him and after finishing cleaning up the kitchen, I wanted to discuss with him what his intentions were. He was determined he wanted us to get married so after our conversation concluded and I made my heart felt apology, I told him he needed to improve his timing and not propose during housework duties. Thankfully, we were still on talking terms.

We rarely went out for dinner as it was not something we could really afford at the time. It was also difficult to make time to go out as Mitchell was only young and as much as my Mum and Dad were there to babysit him whenever possible, they worked full time and it was a one-hour drive to their home. One weekend several weeks after Craig's washing up proposal, my Mum and Dad looked after Mitch for the weekend. We were aware of a lovely seafood restaurant which was in the local shopping centre just a five-minute drive down the road. Neither of us had been so we decided to book a table. It was at this point, during our lovely seafood dinner that the timing was right and Craig proposed without any washing up included. It was a complete turnaround from his first proposal as this was most definitely a romantic night, he got down on one knee in a crowded restaurant and asked if I would marry him. He was very brave. I immediately said "YES" and everyone in the restaurant applauded and cheered for our new engagement. We both agreed that we should get married on Valentine's Day.

CHAPTER 33

# TRAGIC DIAGNOSIS

Shortly after our engagement, Mum noticed some unusual changes in Dad. He could not explain things like he used to be able to. He presented with some kind of confusion over topics that he was always so passionate about and with so much confidence. Mum questioned if it could possibly be a post-traumatic stress symptom after the plane crash and although Mum and Dad discussed Dad's condition, he would simply get up every day and as per usual Mum and Dad would make their journey to work. He was well however he did want to sleep more. This was concerning for Mum as Dad had always gone to bed at about midnight and would wake up bright and early the following day. Dad was always able to live a very healthy life on about six or seven hours sleep per night. After some concern, Mum took Dad to the doctor for a diagnosis of what could possibly be wrong with him. He was still very capable of carrying out any task he put his mind to however it was his thought process and memory that Mum was concerned about.

After many different doctors, tests, and specialist appointments, it was confirmed that my brilliant Dad, a man who was a hero in helping millions of people around the world with his invention, was diagnosed with Alzheimer's. This was a terrible blow for both Mum and Dad although it was a known fact that my Dad's brothers and sisters were also affected by Alzheimer's, it was heartbreaking to find that a man who was so extremely clever and smart would be gradually taken from us with a horrible disease.

Dad was only 67 years of age, and he was looking forward to planning his retirement with Mum. Dad loved his work immensely and he also loved the interaction with his work colleagues. Mum felt the same way so although they knew the time to consider retirement was coming close, they both agreed they would continue to work until they were no longer able to either travel or be physically capable of working full-time.

The news of Dad's condition was something that took quite some adjustment for many months for them both. Mum was concerned that if she mentioned the illness to their friends and work colleagues, they would see Dad in a different light, and this was something that Mum regrettably had to cover up for quite some time. Dad was struggling to come to terms with his recent diagnosis as he had been so academically brilliant his entire life, and he also had extremely good health. His main concern was that he would be a burden on Mum and myself, so in the early stages it was extremely important for Mum and Dad to make solid decisions about their future life, travel, finance, home and of course death. It was crucial for Mum and Dad to make the proper decisions about factors in life that the average person rarely considers during their early to mid-life timeframe. Mum and Dad were concerned that with me being an only child, I would be the one faced with having to make quite emotional and ethical decisions about how and what I needed to do when they were both unable to look after themselves. After considering what plans were needed, Mum, Dad and I saw a solicitor and set in place the necessary paperwork which would enable both Mum and I to make any health or financial decisions relating to Dad's wellbeing.

Mum and Dad made the decision to both continue work at ResMed. Dad was in a happy, safe, and comfortable place at ResMed, not only within the building but also within an environment that made his everyday a place of great respect, friendship, workmanship, and great achievement. Both Mum and Dad spoke with the CEO and made it clear to him that Dad's condition may progress rapidly or it would continue to show small signs of progression. The boss was happy for Dad to continue his work with the company as his work over the many years of his employment were extremely beneficial for the development of the business.

At the time of Dad's employment, the staff observed a very tight knit environment, and everyone involved in the work Dad did was there to make sure he was in a good space both emotionally and mentally. It was decided that the people he worked with would be on hand to monitor Dad's ability to still work at full capability. It was also decided that as his condition progressed, other tasks would be created which would enable Dad to work until he could no longer continue.

CHAPTER 34

# A PERFECT WEDDING DAY

Our wedding day 14th February 1998 arrived more rapidly than Craig and I could anticipate. We were looking forward to a beautiful wedding on the headland which was directly across the road from Mum and Dads' house. Our backdrop was the Pacific Ocean, so we were really hoping, as most brides do, for a stunning day with blue sky and a gentle breeze. We were hoping for a slight breeze so we could be cooled down and protected from the usual humid conditions February offered in Australia. Thankfully, our wishes for perfect weather were granted. The day was filled with blue skies, a brilliant blue ocean which was calm and peaceful and the breeze we had been so strongly hoping for was enough to keep the heat of the day at a very moderate temperature.

Our wedding was a day neither of us will ever forget. Mitch was our most adorable ringbearer, looking dapper in his little suit. I had made a small silk pillow for him to carry our wedding rings on, the pillow matched the colour of my wedding dress which Craig's Mum made for me. Dress making was her forte so with a specific design in my mind, she set to work, with the assistance of Craig's Dad who was a tailor in his earlier working life, and together they created the most beautiful wedding dress which was champagne in colour and champagne in design.

After a beautiful wedding, we flew to Fiji for our honeymoon. We were lucky to be upgraded to business class on the flight over, our honeymoon on a remote Fiji island was beyond any holiday either of us had experienced. I had been to England and Europe in my earlier years and Craig had travelled to Norfolk Island and within Australia, so our Fiji trip was a very different experience from what we were used to. The laid-back atmosphere at the resort was very relaxing and the staff were the friendliest and happiest people we had ever met. The weather, although very hot, was something we were thankful for as we would get stunningly beautiful sunny days followed by a very quick shower in the afternoons which cooled everything down.

CHAPTER 35

# THE NEXT STAGE

After we returned from our honeymoon, we settled into married life very quickly. Mitchell had just started school and we both had discussed having a baby. I had fully disclosed to Craig the real possibility of not being able to provide him with a baby due my antibody condition. He understood to a point the difficulty I faced not being able to carry a baby without my blood destroying the foetus however he did not really understand the actual details of the condition, so we decided to make an appointment with a haematologist.

This was a specialist who knew exactly about blood and could explain to Craig what my blood group and antibodies would do to any possible future pregnancies that I may have. Prior to our appointment, she gave Craig a referral for a blood test. This was apparently important as although she was fully aware of my blood type and antibodies, she had no idea what Craig's blood type or group was. Craig's blood results would give her the information she needed to help us understand the probability of having a baby, with or without the complications of my antibodies. On arrival at the appointment with the haematologist, we both felt very comfortable with her welcoming nature. We also felt like we were in very good hands as she would provide us with the necessary information which would hopefully enable us to move forward in our decision to have a baby.

It was important for me to do whatever I could to carry a baby for a second pregnancy as I was blessed with a boy however, at the age of almost forty,

Craig had not been lucky enough to father a child up to this time in his life. He was extremely close with his little mate Mitch, and he adored him and loved him as his own son, however it was something sitting in the back of my head telling me that not only would I love another baby, but I wanted Craig to have his blood line carried on through future generations.

After the test results for Craig arrived, we were thankfully given the information by the haematologist that Craig's blood group and type would give the two of us a fifty percent chance of producing a baby with a negative blood group. This was the happiest news we could have received, this meant that I had half a chance of giving birth to a baby with blood that was compatible with mine and therefore my antibodies would not cause any problems during pregnancy and certainly would not be detrimental to our unborn baby if the baby's blood were negative.

## CHAPTER 36

# WELCOME BUT CONCERNING NEWS

We both tempted fate in making the decision of producing a baby with a negative blood group and at the beginning of 1999, we were blessed with the news that I was pregnant. Due to my previous complications with my first pregnancy, I was very closely monitored by the Obstetrician which entailed a fortnightly blood test. I made the right decision to see the same Obstetrician I saw during my pregnancy with Mitchell as he was fully aware of my medical condition, not only with the antibodies but also diabetes. I felt comfortable with him, and I knew that even though it had been almost seven years prior, I was confident that he would use the same team of professionals that he used during my last pregnancy and birth. It was the same great team of doctors that allowed me to safely give birth to my baby boy.

Very early in my second pregnancy rhesus antibodies showed a presence in my blood test, this confirmed that our unborn baby's blood was positive. Craig's blood group was positive and although we took our chances to produce a negative blood group baby, it was clear that we were now on a long, stressful road over the next few months. A baby with positive blood would mean that my blood would see it as a foreign body and naturally try to destroy it.

Craig was really concerned, and I was petrified as I had been through a similar situation at the end of my pregnancy with Mitchell, so I was fully aware of what I was going to experience over the next few months. Also, the thought of losing my baby at the end of such a high-risk pregnancy was painfully exhausting for both of us mentally and physically. I was aware that during an amniocentesis there would be a major risk of miscarriage, and I knew that I would require several of them during my pregnancy with our new baby.

Approximately mid-way through my pregnancy I was informed that my antibody level was far too high for the baby to survive too much longer in the womb. It was suggested that I have an amniocentesis and depending on the results, I would possibly require an intrauterine blood transfusion. The sound of this made me shudder with fear, not only due to the invasive procedure but also the fear of what such a procedure could do to my unborn baby. Very shortly after the amniocentesis was carried out, the results were available and it was with these results that made it very clear to both of us that if we decided not to go ahead with the intrauterine blood transfusion, our baby would struggle to survive. Our hearts were racing, and our heads were spinning as we listened to the finer details of the procedure I was about to endure. It was explained to us that they would transfer blood from a compatible doner via a very long and thick needle into my tummy via ultrasound and then inject it into the umbilical cord. This would then be a way to allow my baby to benefit from the compatible blood from the donor.

As the day arrived for the procedure to happen, I was admitted to the maternity section of the hospital and was to be kept there for monitoring for the next couple of days. As I am normally not a very good patient, I was extremely nervous and anxious about what I was about to be faced with. This was a procedure I had never even heard about, let alone be the one that required it.

Craig and I were taken to another part of the hospital, we went to the basement floor of the maternity section, escorted by a team of mostly curious members from the blood bank together with hospital staff. We were taken to a room at the end of a very long corridor which was only lit up by fluorescent lighting on the ceiling. There were absolutely no windows, so the journey was a little depressing for both of us. Thankfully, the medical team were very aware of my fear and concerns, so they were all very friendly and were making me laugh at the funny things they said. The banter between them all was extremely funny and comforting which helped me deal better with what I was about to embark on.

On arriving to the procedure room, we were confronted with another team of doctors and nurses. It was at this point that my fear increased as I could now understand that the intrauterine blood transfusion was not going to be a simple or ultra-safe procedure. The full procedure was explained to us and thankfully Craig was there with me to hold my hand and experience with me what was about to happen.

It was of great importance that I continuously checked my sugar levels as I could not allow the stress of what I was going through affect my baby. The doctors were aware of my extremely tight control, as well as the fact that my Dad had invented the world's first home blood glucose tester, so they therefore allowed me to monitor my own sugar levels and I reported every test I did so they could write the reading on my medical records.

I was given a local anaesthetic in my pregnant tummy and after a few minutes, the procedure began. I was petrified at this stage as the needle was as long as a ruler, simply seeing it was psychologically pain enough. Just the thought of it made my head spin and with a needle this big, I certainly did not want to move in case the needle got my baby. The intrauterine blood transfusion was carried out under very tight monitoring. There was an ultrasound being done at the same time which would allow the specialist to make sure the needle was going into the correct spot of the umbilical cord.

Both Craig and I were able to view the monitor and we watched the entire procedure unfold in front of our eyes. It certainly was not pain free however my main fear was that I would move at the time the needle entered the umbilical cord, so I tried hard not to move but at the same time I needed to be relaxed for the procedure to be successful. As the needle was positioned, it was slowly and carefully moved into the umbilical cord before the donor blood was administered. All was going well, and our eyes were glued to the monitor as the procedure unfolded. Then the unthinkable happened, my unborn baby had kicked the needle out of the umbilical cord with great force. It was at this stage I knew that we had a little fighter on our hands and although we were petrified the procedure would be unsuccessful, we both knew that without the fight my baby would not survive, so our confidence was boosted.

Watching this all happen on the monitor was simply amazing. We were able to see what we thought was "fairy dust" falling out of the needle point which although in black and white, it was a spectacular vision and seemed magical. After they removed the needle from my tummy, we were informed that the baby did not get the total amount of blood that was required due to the fact the needle had been kicked by the baby. They would continue to monitor me closely to see if a second intrauterine blood transfusion would be required. I was sent home the following day and required weekly blood tests at this stage. I was about 25 weeks pregnant so the Obstetrician booked me in for two steroid injections which would help my babies lungs develop. As the next few weeks went by, my pregnancy was just a matter of taking one day at a time. My blood test results would determine when my baby needed to be born and if my antibody levels went much higher, it would not be safe to keep my baby in utero. Every week seemed to drag on as we waited for every result with the greatest of trepidation.

At week 29, my blood test results showed a slight increase in my antibody level so it was decided by my Obstetrician that I would be booked in for a caesarean section at 30 weeks. The baby would not be able to cope with a dangerously high antibody level. It was going to be touch and go either way, so we made the decision to go ahead with what the medical team suggested, after all, it was the same team that delivered Mitchell safely exactly seven years earlier.

Prior to admission to the maternity ward, I decided to have an epidural so I could see my newborn baby take their first breath after the caesarean procedure. I had missed witnessing Mitchell's birth as I thought it would be best to be knocked out completely as I do not deal with pain very well. It was my biggest regret not being able to watch him breathe for the first time, so I decided I did not want to miss out on such an emotion again.

The epidural went without a hitch and within a few minutes, the Obstetrician entered the operating theatre and prepared to begin the surgery. Craig was prepared to be with me every step of the way standing behind me and holding my hand. The surgeon started cutting the lower part of my tummy and I let out an incredibly ear-piercing scream. The Obstetrician stopped what he was doing and took a very prompt step back from the operating table and informed everyone in the theatre that he could no longer carry on with the operation. I was feeling severe pain where he was cutting and the medical team in the birthing unit were aware at this stage that the epidural had not worked. He noticed on making his initial cut through my tummy that the muscle went into spasm. This meant that I could feel the cut and the intense pain I felt was the reason for my ear-piercing scream. He immediately requested that Craig should leave the operating theatre as at that point the caesarean became an emergency procedure.

Thankfully, my Mum and Dad were waiting patiently in the hospital maternity ward with Mitchell when they were suddenly joined by Craig who looked white and had tears in his eyes. Mum and Dad were heartbroken as they thought either our baby or I may not have made it. One of the nurses explained to Mum and Dad what had happened, and Craig waited with them for a while as the anaesthetist and doctor very promptly administered me with a general anaesthetic. Shortly after, the same nurse returned and took Craig back to the operating theatre to see the birth of our baby.

# CHAPTER 37

# THE ANXIOUS ARRIVAL

On 29th July 1999, at 2.12pm, Craig and I were blessed with the birth of a beautiful baby girl Madison Jayne. She was tiny and weighed only 1.7 kgs however she was perfect in every way. She was immediately rushed to the neonatal intensive care unit, the same place where Mitchell was so well cared for seven years before. I was confident they would do everything possible to make sure our baby girl's health would improve and be able to come home when she was strong enough to start life with her new family. Madison was very small and sick however I was extremely confident that she would improve reasonably rapidly as she had strong spirit and fight in her. Remembering that during the intrauterine blood transfusion Madison had kicked the needle out of the umbilical cord so we were hoping that her fight would continue and we would be welcomed home with us within a few months.

The next several weeks were extremely tough for all of us emotionally. Madison would have some good days and then some extremely bad days. A week after her birth she required a blood transfusion and that is when she started to gradually improve. Thankfully, she was now gaining weight as she was being tube fed with my expressed milk. This continued for a few weeks and although her health was greatly affected from the antibodies, she used the fight that she had in her little soul and continued to improve every day. By this time, I was able to give her plenty of cuddles as she had passed the critical stage which meant she was able to escape from the enclosure of the humidicrib on occasion. I was full of happiness and thanks for the incredible professional work the team of doctors and specialists had carried out during my pregnancy. For me to hold tiny little Madison in my arms was a dream come true and something I thought would never happen. I was an extremely happy Mum and although I had experienced so much concern with both my pregnancies, I was blessed with both a boy and a girl. Mitchell and Craig would visit as often as possible however it was an hour's drive from our home to the hospital and with Craig at work and Mitchell at school, their visits were extremely difficult to organise.

I would visit Madison every day and this made me feel like a commuter to a job as Craig would drop me at the train station and I would travel to the hospital again, as I did when Mitch was born. I carried an esky which contained my expressed milk to make the one-hour trip on the train to the hospital. It had been nearly six weeks since my caesarean operation, so I was due to be given the go ahead from the Obstetrician to be able to drive again. I certainly could not wait for this day to arrive as the train trips were starting to take their toll on me and in turn, this was somehow affecting my milk supply. Just prior to my six-week check-up, we were told we would be able to take baby Madison home within the next week. This was extremely exciting news as it would finally mean that our family of four could look forward to life together.

## CHAPTER 38

# LOCATION CHANGE

As we all adjusted to our new family of four, it was now time for Dad to retire as he had just turned 70 years of age. It came at a time when Mum and Dad had decided to sell their house on the Northern Beaches and move closer to where I lived on the Central Coast of NSW. I was the only one that could help Mum with Dad as his condition had deteriorated to a point where his care needs had greatly intensified. As a family, we decided the best option was for them to move closer to me. Having a family of my own meant I was heavily involved with Mitch at school and Madi at preschool, Craig and I had our own business which kept us busy. Thankfully, the business was very successful and the thought of having to move the kids and the business closer to Mum and Dad was out of the question. It was several other challenges that would make Mum and Dad moving close to us a much easier decision.

Mum and Dad owned quite a magnificent home at Warriewood Beach which was set across three different levels. It was on the crest of a very busy coast road, and it was a steep block of land at the rear of the block. The maintenance of the house and property was becoming too much for Dad and Mum was concerned that leaving Dad at home by himself with his condition could possibly lead to something going wrong, based on the house and its location. Not only was it on a busy road but also being across the road from a sea cliff was a major concern for both Mum and I. Although the views across the Pacific Ocean were absolutely stunning, it may present problems if Dad, in future years, was to walk across the busy road or find himself lost.

Mum and Dad decided on the real estate agent they would use to sell their home. It was suggested by the agent that as the property was perfectly positioned in a location which offered stunning views, they should auction their home. At that time, there was a lifestyle television show running called Location Location Location. The producers of that show had approached Mum and Dad's real estate agent to see if it would be possible having the whole sales process, together with the actual auction day made into an episode of the show. Mum and Dad decided that it would be ok for television cameras to cover the sales process of their property. Leading up to the auction there was plenty of interest, open house day was always on a Saturday and became very busy with both perspective buyers and members of the television show, all fighting for space in the house.

As auction day fast approached, Mum and I spent many hours preparing and staging the house for not only the auction but also to be fabulously presented for the television show. The weather was spectacular on auction day and the view from the front of the property presented a stunning backdrop for the big event. There were several bidders which included a well-known sports star. Although the auction began slowly, the bidding got close to the set reserve. Bidding then stopped and the auctioneer thought that as the final offer was so close to the reserve price, placing it on the market may stir up further interest from the bidders. Mum gave the ok to put the house on the market and as the auctioneer predicted, the auction moved forward very quickly, and the offers continued to rise. The final offer was taken, and the property was sold which now meant that Mum and Dad needed to find another home reasonably quickly.

Mum and Dad spent many days with me house hunting for a property on the Central Coast of NSW that would be suitably located close to all the medical facilities and shops. It was also a necessity for them to find a house that Dad could accommodate not only them both but also a house or property that would fit all his bits and bobs that he had collected over the years.

After several weeks of constant searching, Mum and Dad found a home that was on two and a half acres of land. It was a stunning property located a very short distance to all the requirements they needed. It was close to a large shopping centre, a small grocery store, medical facilities, as well as a short drive to Terrigal Beach. Mum loved seeing the ocean and although buying another home near the beach was not something they wanted, it was important for Mum to be close enough to visit the ocean from time to time. There were also some lovely restaurants and clubs in the area surrounding the home, so it was ticking most of the boxes. The property had been on the market for quite some time and from what I understand, no offers had been made.

After a thorough inspection of the home, Mum was concerned that it felt old inside and certainly needed a few minor alterations to make it a comfortable and welcoming home for them both. It was single level, and the rooms were large and open. It was complimented with 9-foot ceilings and a large, covered veranda which surrounded the entire home. It was a solid brick home with great potential and Mum was comfortable in knowing that with the minor adjustments and a coat of paint, the house would be more than suitable for their needs.

Dad was a hoarder of all things, and he was always extremely precise in how he would store and look after his tools, machinery, and equipment. I suggested that I arrange to have a large shed built to accommodate all of Dad's possessions. Although Dad's health was deteriorating, his mind thankfully continued to allow him to create tinker and repair, so it was extremely important to Mum and I that Dad continue this enjoyment.

Mum and Dad decided to put an offer on the property and thankfully, within a very short timeframe, the owners agreed to Mum and Dad's offer. Settlement was the usual six weeks, so we asked for a slightly longer settlement and to be able to access the property to make the necessary alterations which included new flooring throughout, painting throughout and new window dressings.

As the owners of the property had moved out several months prior, they were happy for us to make the necessary changes to the home before settlement and that arrangement was included in the contract. As Mum and Dad were still living in their home on the northern beaches, it was easier and more convenient for me to oversee all the alterations in their new home, that also meant that Mum would have the excitement of seeing the improvements for the first time after settlement. This gave her something to really look forward to and she was once again in mixed emotions for fear of making a wrong move and hoping they had made the right decision. The huge job of packing up their old home was a concern for Mum on how the move would affect Dad. His condition was deteriorating fast, and it was at this stage that Mum knew that the sorting, packing and moving would be basically done by herself with very limited help from Dad.

Dad was now getting very confused with where things belonged and how to stack or store them. This certainly was not going to be an easy task for Mum as she was finding that whatever she packed was frustratingly being unpacked and placed elsewhere by Dad. Mum had methods that worked extremely well for her during her packing and although Dad was aware that they were to be moving in a short period of time, he could not quite comprehend that the packed boxes were to be left alone and stored ready for moving day.

Mum considered paying for a removal company to pack their entire belongings however with Dad's fragile equipment and machinery, together with Mum's special collection of ornaments, Mum thought it was best for her to go through items and decide what was needed and wanted to be kept and what could be thrown out. She also based her decision on Dad's condition as she knew that Dad would at some stage require further medical assistance, whether it was going to be at home or in a nursing home. This was an extremely sad and cruel unknown. Mum was wanting to save whatever money she could to put towards their retirement years and she felt that the packing was something she could do herself. She did not want to waste any of their hard-earned savings.

Days of packing and sorting out their belongings turned into weeks of hard work as Dad continued his process of unpacking different objects and items from boxes that prompted memories for him. So sad to watch his brain slowly diminish as he had always been so sharp and confident with knowledge and total understanding. It was a torturous job for Mum as she knew that she was packing their belongings that included a lifetime of memories. It prompted thoughts that she was packing items that Dad would no longer have any recollection of or use for and this is what made the task of packing an extremely emotional time for Mum. She knew that it would not be too long before Dad was not able to remember any of wonderful memories shared together during their decades of marriage.

As Mum continued her packing, I was making good progress at their new home. The painting was completed, and the new flooring and window coverings were about to be installed. The house was certainly looking much brighter, and I was content that Mum and Dad would be able to move into a home that would be fresh and clean and ready for their new life chapter, and she would not have to expose Dad to any disruptive work within the house once they had moved in.

I had also proposed to the local council permission to build a shed large enough for all of Dad's tools, equipment, and machinery. Thankfully, the shed was quickly approved and once again this was included in the contract for the sale of the property. It was important for both Mum and I that Dad would be able to utilise his new shed as soon as possible after moving. We knew that his shed was his happy place, and he could tinker for hours every day by doing what he loved.

It was settlement day for both properties and this was a bittersweet day for my Mum. She was about to leave the house that she had lived in for so long and loved so much, her house with a stunning view of the Pacific Ocean and many fabulous memories. She was also sad to leave her Sydney friends and neighbours and moving to a new house and a new area was quite emotional for her. Dad was at the stage of his illness where he was not fully aware of what they were about to encounter so he happily went along with whatever the day brought. Mum and Dad settled quite quickly into their new home and as it was single level, Mum found it much easier to live in. Both homes that they previously owned after their arrival in Australia were double storey, so they were both happy that their new home did not have any stairs this time. It was also a blessing for Mum as Dad was now starting to wander and it was important for her to know that he was safe without the very strong possibility of him falling down any stairs.

CHAPTER 39

# THE NOT-SO-GREAT ESCAPE

Dad was full time for Mum as he was now at the stage where he could not remember very much. He was more and more confused and was now losing his capability of being able to make himself a cup of tea, turn the television on and off, as well as even being able to take himself to the toilet. He would get lost within the house and Mum struggled to be able to have a quick shower without him emptying a cupboard or trying to repair something that Dad felt was broken, even if it were not. Mum and I decided to fit some magnetic door alarms so if Dad tried to open any of the doors, an alarm would sound which would alert Mum immediately. This enabled her to be able to have a shower without worrying about Dad opening a door and taking off somewhere.

Mum was constantly run off her feet trying to keep Dad within a safe and happy environment so the fitting of alarms for the doors was a necessary requirement. The magnetic alarms worked perfectly, and they would alert Mum if Dad were to open any of the doors in preparation to walk outside and possibly onto the road or even into the dam which was located at the bottom of the property. Mum was concerned that Dad would get run over on the main road which was a major thoroughfare between the two main highways on the Central Coast of NSW. The road was only one lane in each direction without a pedestrian footpath which made it dangerous for anyone walking beside the road. It was approximately 300 feet from the house however my Dad loved to walk and as he was still extremely physically fit, he was still capable of walking so it was inevitable that he would venture down to the road and possible be hit by a car. This was also the case with the dam. Dad loved the dam on the property as he would watch the ducks and turtles enjoy the water and the dam environment. He would stand at the kitchen window and watch the dam for hours. It was a forever changing scene which kept Dad occupied on a regular basis.

Mum was concerned that if he walked down to the pond and slipped or fell, he would not be able to comprehend how to get out of the water. Both Mum and I were concerned as the dam was his favourite place on the property it would only be a matter of time before this happened. We were both extremely concerned that if this were to happen during any time Mum took her eyes off Dad's whereabouts, he would open the door and visit his favourite spot.

Within a few months of installing the very successful and reliable magnetic alarms, Mum always made sure Dad was comfortable watching one of his favourite movies on the television. Dad had always loved war movies and his fascination for planes and history had been very important to him since he was a little boy. He would sit for hours re watching The Great Escape. He was enthralled in the movie every time he watched it, and it was a guarantee for Mum that Dad was not getting into any danger while he sat and watched in awe such a great movie.

It would give Mum time to hang washing out, have a shower, cook dinner, any routine requirements were carried out by Mum with forward planning and strategic thinking as to what Dad could get up to. She needed to constantly make sure that Dad was safe and could in no way hurt himself. Thinking ahead is something that Mum became good at, more so now than before Dad became sick. She had made sure Dad was enthralled with watching his favourite movie and decided to have a quick shower. This one specific occasion Mum had showered and got dressed and came out to discover that Dad had somehow escaped the safety of the house. She was confused as she would always hear the alarm sound if any door were opened. She did not hear anything on this occasion, and it was always at the back of her mind that if any of the doors were opened, she would hear an ear-piercing sound which would immediately alert her.

With immediate panic and concern, Mum searched the house to see if Dad was still inside. Their house was quite a large and very long home and Mum practically ran from one room to the next looking for Dad. Within a frantic minute or two, Mum realised that Dad had opened one of the doors and set off extremely quickly. He had managed to turn the television off, which was a task that he normally struggled with. He then disconnected and pulled apart the magnetic door alarm. He had dismantled the entire mechanism. This is sadly where we knew that somewhere sometimes deep down, my Dad's brain was still very capable. He had gone through the kitchen drawers looking for a screwdriver and once he had found what he was looking for, he very meticulously dismantled the alarm without damaging it or causing any destruction of the door or door frame.

Mum was in a major state of panic at this stage as she knew that he could be anywhere, especially as he was very fit and although he did not go to a gymnasium or lift weights, he had always looked after his health so his ability to walk very quickly was certainly something of which he was quite capable. Mum immediately contacted the police and explained to them the situation and details about my Dad's appearance, together with information about where their home was located. Mum then immediately asked the neighbours if they had seen Dad and unfortunately, they were unable to give her the news for which she was hoping. The neighbours went in different directions in their cars to see if they could find him. Mum was extremely reluctant to contact me as she knew that any stress could and possibly would affect my sugar levels. She did not want me to be worried or concerned so therefore made the decision not to contact me for a couple of hours after Dad's disappearance. She finally decided that it was time to contact me, and I knew immediately when she spoke to me on the phone that there was something wrong. I was really concerned about what news she was about to inform me of and just by listening to the quiver in her voice, I knew it was not going to be good news.

Through Mum's stammering and hesitation, it took Mum some time to let me know that Dad was missing. It had been a couple of hours by this stage so when she told me the timing of his disappearance, I remembered a family friend who went missing and never returned. I could not stop thinking about this and was extremely fearful that due to his loss of basic cognitive skills, my Dad may never be found alive.

The local area surrounding Mum and Dad's home consisted of mostly farm properties and a school precinct. The area was also surrounded by dense bushland, dams, roads with no footpaths and adding another deadly aspect to this scenario, the weather was getting extremely cold, it was the middle of winter. It was incredible wondering how Dad, in his current state, would be able to deal with any situation he may be faced with during his wilful desire to adventure.

Within a few hours, Mum received a phone call from the police. Amazingly my Dad had been found. He had ventured from his home, along a main road without a footpath, across a four-lane highway and then taken a detour via a quiet backstreet which had several houses. The backstreet then led to another main road, and it was off this road, in a small cul-de-sac, where a lady was watering her garden. Dad had stopped to admire her garden as he was always amazed at the beauty that mother nature could offer. The garden that he had stopped to look at grabbed his interest which was to be a blessing in disguise. The lady watering her plants noticed Dad had stopped to look at her garden and she thought it was slightly odd that a man in his mid-70's would be holding an old hessian bag.

As she lived close to a retirement village, she felt the man had wandered off from the safe surrounds of the nearby nursing home, she asked him if he would like a cup of tea. A cup of tea was my Dad's favourite drink. He knew he liked milk and no sugar so when asked how he preferred his tea, he promptly replied with milk but no sugar. He was also offered a piece of apple pie which was my Dad's favourite dessert. The lady then offered him a seat in her loungeroom and continued to try to find out where Dad had come from before contacting the police. She asked Dad his name and immediately he answered "Stan Clark, Clark without the E" This was how Dad had always said his name when he introduced himself.

The lady then asked him what the hessian bag was about, and he mentioned that he had found it for his mother. My Dad's Mum was a dear old beautiful woman whom he absolutely adored so something in my Dad's poor unwell mind was creating a memory of his mother. It was at this stage that the caring lady that was so very curious about my Dad's appearance, became fully aware that Dad was unwell mentally. After making sure Dad was happy with his tea and apple pie, she contacted the police to give them whatever information she could about my Dad and the conversation she just had with him. It was shortly after she made the call to the police that Mum was informed that Dad had been found safe and well and immediately Mum and Dad's neighbour drove Mum to pick Dad up from the lady with the beautiful garden. Mum and I, today still reminisce about the time Dad went wandering and the fabulous lady that quite possibly saved his life. It was extremely lucky as dense bushland was near where the lady found Dad and if he had wandered in the wrong direction, he may have perished.

## CHAPTER 40

# BUILT WITH LOVE

It was shortly after this time that I realised my Mum could no longer look after Dad at home. Mum was becoming weak both physically and emotionally and I was very concerned that it would not be long before I lost them both if Mum didn't get her own mind space to be able to function properly herself. My Dad was now requiring 24-hour care and Mum was struggling with Dad's everyday needs. It was important that she maintained his love of the simple things in life, which he so passionately enjoyed.

It was at this stage it was necessary for me to fully utilise the abundance of land that Mum and Dad lived on. During my growing years, Dad had always spoken to me about dual occupancy. It simply meant that two groups of people or family could live together on the same property. I have absolutely no idea why this was something that Dad had discussed with me however it was at this stage that I felt a very strong desire to investigate his dual occupancy theory more closely. After further investigation into this, I decided that it would be the only way forward as Mum could keep Dad at home much longer. The property was becoming too much work for Dad, and he simply was not capable of looking after it himself. It was a large block of land together with a very large home, hired help was the order of the day for gardening and lawns and general maintenance which was a daily requirement. Dad also sometimes had the help of Craig and Mitchell however the huge cost of hired help was becoming unrealistic.

Dad had always pleaded with Mum to keep him at home and not put him into full time care. This was always something that Mum had promised would not happen. Mum and I had many discussions that the time may possibly come when she was no longer able to look after Dad within their own home. Mum was able to get small amounts of help around the house from paid carers. The carers would also come and sit with Dad to allow Mum to get her housework and washing done however the care that Dad required was becoming more and more intense.

After several months of planning, we had decided on the best design of a second house for the property. With very prompt approval from the local council, I supervised having a home built on Mum and Dad's behalf. This home was purposely designed for Mum to be able to better look after Dad in the safest possible way. The home was to be open plan, single level living with easy access from one room to another, without long hallways. It contained two bedrooms with built in robes, both bedrooms contained an ensuite bathroom. The second bedroom ensuite also doubled as the main bathroom. The kitchen, dining and living areas were all open plan and extremely spacious. The floor to ceiling glass bay window in the dining room would allow sunlight into the entire living area as well as showcasing the beautiful view over the pond. The house also contained a study which could be used as a bedroom if required as well as a storage room.

My husband, my kids and I made a family decision to move into Mum and Dad's existing home on the property, this was a very difficult decision as we had only recently put an upstairs addition on our family home, a home that was also purposely built to suit our family requirements. I was lucky enough to have found a great team of tradesmen to put an extension on our Kariong home so with the same fabulous tradesmen I was able to complete Mum and Dad's new home within four months. I thoroughly enjoyed the project management part of the build, and it was thrilling to see the design that had been swirling around in my head for many sleepless nights, come to fruition.

As Mum and Dad's new home was being built, it was certainly a very exciting spectacle for my Dad to observe, my Dad's health was becoming more and more difficult for Mum to take care of. Thankfully, my Dad was never aggressive which is something that I was concerned about as never in my life had I ever experienced that kind of behaviour from him. Dad always had a gentle and kind way and the thought of him changing his demeanour can often be a developing symptom of people with his illness, this thought was not something with which I could face.

I had always been blessed with a loving, caring, and thoughtful Dad, a Dad that I was very close to. It was my main concern after learning about Dad's illness he would get to a point where he did not remember me. I was aware that people suffering Alzheimer's would eventually lose their ability to remember who someone was, even though they had known them for a very long time. I was fearful that the humble man that had created the most amazing piece of equipment, which not only helped me but helped the future of diabetes sufferers around the world, could possibly forget his only child's existence. This was a heartbreaking reality for me that was a distinct possibility.

# CHAPTER 41

# THE TOUGHEST DECISION

Sadly, prior to Mum and Dad's new home being completed, it was necessary for Dad to be admitted to a nursing home. He was now at the point where it was becoming impossible for him to communicate properly and be understood. Mum was unable to sleep at night, and the strain was debilitating for her. Anyone who has experienced the emotional turmoil of having to make the heart-breaking decision to put their much-loved family member into a nursing home will understand how hard this was, especially as my Dad always put other people's needs before his own. This man who had helped millions of people living with diabetes, together with their family and friends who are affected by someone living with this condition... Absolutely heartbreaking...

Mum and I were lucky enough to find a lovely nursing home which was approximately 15 minutes away from the property Mum and Dad had purchased for their retirement. Mum had a lovely little bright blue car which she absolutely adored so she was happy to visit Dad daily. She also wanted to spend as much time as possible with him because she knew that he had been suffering his illness for several years by now and he would not live for very much longer.

Thankfully, the new home at Holgate had now been completed and Mum was able to move in. Dad's idea of dual occupancy had become a reality, we now had two homes on the Holgate property. I was happy knowing that Mum would not be home alone on the property and within a couple of days of moving Mum into her new place, we moved from my home of 25 years at Kariong into Mum and Dad's original home at Holgate. This meant that the whole family would be closer to the nursing home, so we took every opportunity we had to visit Dad.

We would take items that Dad loved so much to the nursing home to see if it would jog his memory and give him the thrill of being able to possibly remember his great life achievements. We decided to take him one of the first glucose testers he had ever built and thankfully, we were able to sit with him for hours as he pondered with wonder at what he was looking at and touching. We knew that he remembered what he had created yet he was unable to articulate the fact, even though he could not tell us his thoughts, we still felt satisfaction watching his joy inspecting his worldwide creation.

CHAPTER 42

# SAYING GOODBYE TO A HERO

Within three years of Dad moving into the nursing home, we were informed that they did not think Dad was going to make it through the night. Mum and I immediately went to be with him, and we were able to stay with him during his last hours. The nursing home had transferred him to the chapel which was provided with a double sofa bed and several comfortable chairs. The chapel was filled with lots of filtered sunlight which came through the beautiful lead light glass and large picture windows. Through the windows was a view that looked out onto the immaculately manicured gardens surrounding the nursing home. This was very comforting for both Mum and I to know that Dad was in a good place. We stayed with Dad and left only very briefly to get some lunch. We were offered coffee and tea and cold drinks by the wonderful, caring staff at the nursing home, and this is one of the main reasons we had chosen where Dad would spend his last years. Their care and compassion were beyond remarkable and with this, both Mum and I knew that Dad would be in the best hands.

We stayed with Dad overnight and thankfully as we had been provided with a sofa bed, we were both able to manage to get some sleep. Dad was comfortable and thankfully still knew who we both were. At one point he looked directly into my eyes, and I had grown up remembering that look, a look that reassured me of how much he loved and adored me. As heartbreaking as it was to see my Dad possibly look at me for the last time, I felt unconditional love for him when he looked at me this way. I was comforted in knowing that my Dad, even with advanced Alzheimer's, knew who I was until his very last breath.

Both Mum and I went home briefly to have a quick shower and put some clean clothes on. When we returned to the chapel, Dad was still comfortable, yet his conscious state was deteriorating rapidly. We sat with him and told him stories of what we did as a family during our lives together and we constantly let him know that he was the best husband and father that any wife and daughter could ask for. We also told him how much we loved and adored him. We never once said how much we would miss him and how heartbroken we would be when his time came, we did not want Dad to have any negativity or heartbreak in knowing how devastated we were going to be when he passed.

Later that afternoon, as we both held his hand, my beautiful Dad took his last breath. My beautiful father died on the 7$^{th}$ of June 2011. I was inconsolable and Mum was devastated although Mum had spent every day with Dad during his last few years, so she was, over time, slowly preparing for Dad to leave her side. The illness that killed Dad was a genetic condition that ran in his family, an illness that had also killed several of his brothers and sisters.

My two children, Mitchell, and Madison were devastated. They were both extremely close to their Grandad. He was the Grandad that every one of their friends wished they had, he would make things for them as well as show them how to create items for themselves, just like he did for me when I was young. It would be these memories that I hope would stay with them forever. Memories that they will share with their own children in later years. He gave the best cuddles and loved them both unconditionally.

We were grieving the loss of the most adorable and humble human being and proceeded with the emotional task of planning for his funeral. The east Coast of NSW, including Sydney and the Central Coast, was affected by extremely hazardous weather conditions at the time, which I say was the world crying their tears for my Dad. There were thunderstorms, torrential rain, and floods all the way along the east coast of NSW. There were so many people we wanted to invite as they most certainly would not be able to attend

Dad's funeral during this major weather event. The funeral was organised ten days after Dad's death and as hard as the morning was, the clouds parted, and we were blessed with a beautifully bright sunny day for the hundreds of people wanting to say their goodbyes to my Dad. The chapel was set amongst a stunning backdrop of beautiful plants and waterfalls, something my Dad, with his love of mother nature, would have loved.

Dad's funeral was a wonderful celebration of his life, it was a beautiful memorial, the weather, the service, and the wake, all played their part. The day was filled with heartfelt emotion with a hundred plus mourners attending to pay tribute to a very special man, the man that had invented the home blood glucose monitoring system for diabetics, the man that enabled pregnant woman with diabetes to be able to carry a baby to full term, confident with the knowledge that their accurate glucose levels would ensure the safe delivery of their newborn babies. The man that enabled diabetics suffering eye damage from uncontrolled high sugar levels be able to manage their glucose levels at home and repair their eyesight with tight control. My Dad certainly broke the mould with his amazing invention along with his caring, beautiful nature. My Dad was a very special human being, and his legacy will be remembered through future generations.

Over the next few months our family was still in disbelief, our lives were full of emotional upheaval, we were only too painfully aware that we lost a much loved husband, Dad, and Grandad, a man that revolutionised diabetic control and management. Certainly, a man who will never be forgotten by diabetic sufferers and their families, now and in future generations.

CHAPTER 43

# BUILDING NEW MEMORIES

My Mum loved her new home and thankfully she was able to enjoy building her own memories in a place where she never had the experience of living with Dad. It eased the burden in grieving the loss of her husband of nearly 60 years. She was able to move around her new home without any memories of Dad sitting in the loungeroom or sleeping in the bedroom. Although every day was difficult, the new home provided a haven for her without the reminder of Dad having lived in the house.

We were always close by as the two houses were adjoined by an extremely large carport. This would allow us the ability to walk from one house to the other undercover. The houses were also suitable for walker or wheelchair access in case, in the future, Mum would possibly require assistance with her walking. It was a gradual process for Mum to come to terms with her grief however she was now slowly able to enjoy her home but also, she now had the time to be able to reconnect with her friends. My Mum had always been lucky enough to have beautiful friends, she now cherished every moment of being able to go out with them and was always grateful for their companionship. Every one of her friends missed my Dad terribly however they knew that Mum's new home was a perfectly suitable environment for her to enjoy and be comfortable.

# CHAPTER 44

# EXEPTIONAL PROJECT

In 2017, nine years after Mum moved into her new home, I was contacted by Diabetes Australia. They mentioned that they had been approached by a young girl, Lilly Hogan, asking if they could help her with a school project. The project was her year six final assignment, and the subject was called "Night of Notables'. The students had been asked to research a person who had made a notable difference, and with herself having had Type 1 diabetes for many years, it seemed appropriate for Lilly that the project was to be about my Dad, Stan Clark. She believed that my Dad's invention had not only helped her but also helped nearly every diabetic around the world.

I was honoured to be asked if I could help Lilly with her project so with the help of her Mum providing transport for Lilly to get to our place, we would then get together with the necessary information for her to start work on her assignment. We were only an hour away which meant we were able to spend quality time with Lilly and were therefore able to provide her with all the information she needed, and then some!

Mum had kept so much information from the many years of glucose tester manufacturing, so it was important for Mum to give Lilly as much information as possible to make sure she got excellent marks for her project.

Mum was overwhelmed with the information that Lilly had already researched about my Dad. Mum was also very touched by the fact that a young girl who was not even alive during the late 1970s and early 1980s was fully aware that my Dad, Stan Clark, was the one who invented the world's first home blood glucose tester decades prior to her birth. Shortly after Lilly completing her project, I was contacted by her Mum and was informed that Lilly received a 97% mark for her project. Mum and I were delighted with her results and still to this day are thankful for Lilly's passion about my Dad's creation. We remain in contact with Lilly and Viv and look forward to watching Lilly grow into a successful and talented young woman. We also know that her passion and brilliance will enable Lilly to excel in whatever field of work she chooses.

## CHAPTER 45

# A LONG PAINFUL ROAD

Thankfully, the house design that was originally planned for the purpose of Dad in the later years of his Alzheimer's, was very beneficial for my Mum as several years after Dad had passed away, Mum was riddled with excruciating pain throughout her body, in particular her hip. After several appointments with specialists and many x-rays and doctors' visits, it was established that my poor Mum was suffering from severe arthritis and also required a hip replacement. As the months went by and Mums pain increased beyond manageable, my poor Mum took a bad turn and her health deteriorated extremely quickly. She was at the point where she could not keep food down and simply felt like she wanted to end her own life.

I struggled to find answers as to what was making her so sick and it was heartbreaking for me to watch my beautiful Mum go through so much pain and with no improvement at all, even with strong doses of medication. I was at breaking point watching Mum suffer so much sickness and pain that I called an ambulance in the hope that they would be able to help her if she were in hospital. My Mum had seemingly overnight gone from a very strong and powerful woman into a frail little old lady that needed to be pushed around in a wheelchair. It was at this time that I was glad that I had designed the house I built for Mum and Dad with wheelchair access, as sadly it had become a necessity for my poor Mum.

Mum's weight had plummeted to 44 kilograms and after a few days in hospital she was transferred to a private hospital and was thankfully placed under the superb care of a specialist. After three months of intense rehabilitation, Mum was able to come home in a much better state, not only with her health but also her mental frame of mind. She had lived with the pain for so long and sadly, the pain is what was making her feel like she had no hope of recovering and no relief from the pain. The specialist altered her medications and together with physiotherapy, Mum was in a much better place. She had been told that she required a hip replacement however although she had gained weight during the three months of rehabilitation, she still was not strong enough to go through the surgical invasion of a hip replacement. After leaving the constant care of rehabilitation, it was now my job to build Mum up so she would be strong enough to endure a hip operation.

Thankfully, the fabulous specialist not only altered her medications but arranged physiotherapy together with giving Mum the psychological hope she needed to get better. He was also responsible for bringing my Mum back to her normal bright self. She could laugh again and was now able to joke, watching my Mum have hope again is something that I will be forever grateful. It was also the specialist's team of carers and medical staff that will be remembered not only by my Mum and myself but our extended family and friends. For the next six months, now Mum was home again, it was my mission to get some additional weight on her so she could survive the surgery and be strong enough to come out the other end without too many concerns.

Growing up with diabetes, I was fully aware of food groups, carbohydrates, fats etc so I knew that I could increase Mum's weight safely, without harming her health. I would make her smoothies; give her yogurt and I would try to feed her with my cooking as often as possible. My Mum had always had a great appetite until the time she became sick. It had become such a struggle what to feed her as she often would not have any appetite at all. At this stage I was left with no other option but to try several different frozen meals. This would enable Mum to choose whatever she wanted at the time and I made sure I ordered healthy options of packaged dinners, I was hopefully confident that she would be getting a balanced diet.

12 months after Mum had been admitted to the emergency ward, with a alarming weight of 44 kilograms, Mum had now increased her weight to a healthy 55 kilograms and was ready both mentally and physically to deal with a hip replacement. Mum was lucky to have a very caring and understanding hip specialist and we both felt we were extremely lucky to once again find another specialist that had so much empathy and expertise to help Mum walk properly again. She was booked in for her hip replacement two weeks later and although I was worried sick that I could possibly lose her, I was confident that she was in excellent hands with her specialist.

On 21st September 2021, Mum and I went to the private hospital not too far from our home. Mum's operation was booked in for 3pm so thankfully we weren't in any rush to get Mum there early. It would take quite some time to get Mum ready as the pain in her hip was still quite unbearable which made getting dressed quite a task. The specialist allowed me to stay until Mum was taken into the operating theatre, and this was actually a very special time for us as while we waited, we had some very deep and meaningful conversations seemingly reconnecting us in a way we never had before. Although I now have my husband and children, during my childhood and adolescent years I grew up with only my Mum and Dad, the three of us, we were a tight, loving family unit and only had each other to depend on and trust. Losing Dad was a major part of our lives and now that family unit was reduced to just the two of us, all I had was my Mum and being able to spend such quality time with her meant the world to me.

As Mum was taken into the operating theatre, I left the hospital and returned home. This was during the Covid pandemic, so I was unable to stay at the hospital during Mum's operation. I was in a reasonable amount of emotional turmoil when I walked out of the hospital, I was happy that Mum would hopefully be free from the pain of her hip however, I was concerned that she possibly would not make it through the operation. She had been so sick for so long and although she was now fitter and much healthier, I was aware that it was a major operation and at the age of eighty-three, anything could go wrong. I had asked the staff to call me when the operation was over and was in recovery. I just wanted to make sure she was OK. I waited for four stressful hours before the phone finally rang. I was in a state of shock, on the other end of the phone, my Mum's voice calmly informed me that she had just had a sandwich and was watching her favourite TV show. I was gobsmacked. My beautiful Mum had not only survived a hip replacement, but she was cohesive and was able to talk to me. My emotions were extremely raw and had been causing low sugar levels so after hearing my Mums bright and cheerful voice, I could now relax somewhat knowing that Mum had come through the operation with flying colours. Within a couple of hours of receiving the phone call from Mum, my sugar levels returned to normal, and I was content knowing that Mum was in good hands and would now be able to begin her recovery by once again going to the original rehabilitation facility.

Mum was transferred to rehabilitation five days after her hip replacement. She spent two weeks with intense physiotherapy and once again she was treated with real care and compassion. She had been through almost three years of intense pain and sickness, and I was certainly happy to know that after all her suffering, she was now on a very positive road to a great recovery.

Within three weeks after my Mum's hip replacement, she returned home with transitional care provided by the hospital. They were going to make sure that her progress was thoroughly maintained through intense physiotherapy and nursing care for her surgical wound. Mum was now reasonably able to manage the pain herself, she was required to continue with her exercises and needed to be particularly careful with her movement for the next few months. She continued to use her walker which enabled her to move around her home with stability and safety.

As the months went by, Mum's improvement was remarkable. She was enjoying her food; she was walking extremely well, and she was now pain free. Her quality of life returned to the same as it was before her illness. Her weight continued to increase, and she could now enjoy life again. Once again, I was extremely thankful to the fabulous specialist and medical teams involved with my Mum's surgery and rehabilitation.

After many years of worrying that my Mum's life force was diminishing, I was able to breathe a sigh of relief knowing that my Mum would thankfully be with us for many more years to come. Mum was now walking with the assistance of a walking stick however she still, to this day, uses her walking stick purely for the confidence it provides. She is now able to wander around her home without any walking aids at all and after years of watching her suffer, I feel extremely thankful that my Mum can enjoy her later years with absolutely no pain or sickness. She is currently 85 years of age and is in good health.

## CHAPTER 46

# A FABULOUS JOURNEY

Today, my children Mitchell and Madison lead very different but successful lives. I am extremely proud of them both, and I know also just how proud my Dad would be. They both continue to spend as much time as possible with my Mum and thankfully, we are a small but close family. My husband Craig is my backbone. We have been together for over 30 years now and he has always been there during my highs and lows, not only with sugar levels but also in every aspect of my life. As always, we have had our challenges as a family however we will always continue to be very proud and give immense gratitude to my Dad for his incredible invention, allowing blood glucose monitoring to be carried out by the patient in a home environment. This was an invention that was created to give me the ability to manage my glucose levels at home. It was also an invention which became a worldwide phenomenon. An invention that not only helped me safely have two healthy children but also an invention that helped millions of people around the world. It was all done purely out of my Dad's love for me. My Dad was an unsung hero until now as writing this book about his extraordinary invention will place him centre stage and now we can all celebrate his remarkable life. We can certainly be assured that my Dad's legacy will continue through future generations with the management of diabetes.

Insulin was the greatest invention in the world of diabetes – but I believe my Dad runs a very close second with his home blood glucose testing invention. As the world advances in all aspects of new technology, it was my father, a pioneer whose name will go down in all of history for his invention. Stan Clark, a devoted husband, a loving father, also a doting grandfather who was brilliant and talented enough to create one of the world's most important changes in diabetes management. His work will be continued in the advancement of diabetes testing of home blood glucose levels forever, and we will always be thankful that he not only helped me, but he helped millions of people around the world.

**Well done Dad, you are a legend!**

## AWARDS

Over the many years of Dad's dedication and his incredible contribution to the safe and successful management of diabetic control, Dad was awarded many very well-deserved awards.

Dad's awards were endless. He was recognised for his successful invention with many awards, including the Order of Australia Medal for his distinguished service to diabetes in 2001; the inaugural Diabetes Australia (National) Award in 1997: he also featured in the television program What'll They Think of Next, receiving a first-place tie; the Diabetes Australia-NSW Diamond Jubilee Award. He became the inventor of the Year in 1978; he won the Australian Small Business Award in 1981 and, also received a bronze medal at the ninth International Inventors' Convention in Geneva in 1980.

Dad was also acclaimed in two international publications – Great Minds of the 21st Century, published in the United States, as well as the prestigious British Dictionary of International Biography.

## THE STAN CLARK CHAIR

"The Stan Clark Chair in Diabetes in Sydney Medical School (Central) of the University of Sydney was commenced in 2014 and bestowed upon Professor Stephen Twigg. The Chair recognises Prof. Twigg's sustained, passionate leadership in translational research, and education of clinicians, to help optimise clinical care of people with Type 1 diabetes. Steve continues to research utilising technology in Type 1 diabetes such as continuous glucose monitoring to enable people with diabetes to safely manage their glucose levels and help prevent diabetes complications. In recent years, he and his team have undertaken studies in Type 1 diabetes and high-intensity exercise, and other studies of metformin and fenofibrate in Type 1 diabetes funded by Diabetes Australia and/or JDRF and philanthropically including the Stan Clark fund. These collaborative trials occurred in the Charles Perkins Centre, the University of Sydney, and in the Department of Endocrinology in Royal Prince Alfred Hospital Diabetes Centre and were published in the top diabetes journals internationally. He has supervised 16 PhD students directly across the years, many of whom have become leaders in diabetes clinical care, and diabetes research in their own right.

Steve is a past President of the Australian Diabetes Society (ADS) and past Health Professional Vice-President of Diabetes Australia plus an Australian delegate to the International Diabetes Federation World Congress, enabling him to help progress the needs of people with diabetes in their care. He was the only adult Endocrinologist on the first Federal Government Committee to commence roll out nationally of continuous glucose monitoring for people with Type 1 diabetes. He was Chair of the NSW DoH Agency for innovation 2011-2018 in Diabetes and Endocrinology, which developed a e-program for safe glucose care for people with type 1 diabetes in public Hospitals in NSW. He commenced the USyd Masters of Metabolic Health Program including in diabetes for younger doctors and GPs to upskill about Type 1 diabetes care. In 2017, he received the DA-NSW Sir Kempson-Maddox Award for services to the diabetes movement and in 2021 the premier Kellion Award of the Australian Diabetes Society, for his outstanding service, research and education and clinical care support, of people with diabetes. Most recently he has commenced research part funded by DA to explore the Kellion Victory medallists (who have had diabetes for 50 years or more) to better support quality of life and longevity in aging in people with Type 1 diabetes.

Steve has a special friendship with Lisa (the author!) and her mother Audrey, and he is highly appreciative of the fundraising that has occurred to date to support his and his team's research.

People interested in supporting the legacy and memory of Stan Clark, and in meeting Prof. Stephen Twigg or funding his research through the Stan Clark Chair, can contact the University of Sydney including the Development Office:

https://www.sydney.edu.au/engage/give/contact-the-donor-support-team.html

## REFLECTIONS

"For most of the 1970s and for decades prior, people with insulin requiring diabetes could only monitor glucose levels by urine tests at home. This was a big problem as urine testing always lags well behind blood tests and it is often a very poor, unreliable reflection of current blood glucose, making dosing with insulin and avoiding severe low blood glucose, highly problematic.

The advent of the first portable blood glucose meter for regular home usage, by Electronics Engineer Mr Stan Clark, was the biggest revolution in aiding safe care of people with diabetes who needed to receive insulin treatment. It was made for his daughter Lisa Harris (back then, Clark), and for other people with diabetes in the later 1970s – as the quote goes, 'for love, not money'. Stan made the first such device in Australia and arguably in the world. For the first time it enabled people with diabetes, and their carers, to confidently measure their blood glucose at home, promptly, reliably, and accurately. Generations of people with diabetes benefitted from self-monitoring of blood glucose, using initially Stan's reflectance glucose meter, then subsequently meters by biotech industry with refined versions that later needed less blood sample and were more rapid.

When people who have had insulin requiring diabetes across the last 50 years or more are asked what the most helpful aid to their care has been, they say the ability to measure blood glucose with a portable meter (Stan's and then other's). In recent years, only other comparable aids to people with diabetes are those in the more modern era of the new millennium with continuous glucose meters and low glucose alarms, sometimes as part of an artificial pancreas system.

It is remarkable then that accessible, portable, accurate glucose sensing has made such a great improvement in quality of life for people with insulin requiring diabetes and has helped to prevent severe low glucose and prevent long term complications of diabetes from otherwise arising due to high average glucose. Thank you to Stan Clark for his revolutionary glucose testing method which advanced the diabetes field so many years and helped so many people."

**Professor Stephen M. Twigg**...*Stan Clark Chair in Diabetes, and current Kellion Professor of Endocrinology 30$^{th}$ May 2022*

Rhonda (my sister) spoke to me today about me sharing some of my memories, back 45 years ago when the infamous Stan Clark invented his blood machine, and the impact it had on my life.

Wow what a life changer.

You see back in the day, I had to borrow my endocrinologist's blood machine for a week at a time, just to see what my BSLs were doing. My family couldn't afford to pay, nor do I think it was available to buy what my specialist had.

All I had at home were the test tubes and clinitest tablets – remember if you held the test tube after putting so many drops of water then urine in the test tube then 1 clinitest tablet, it became very hot. My fingers were often burnt until my dad made me a frame with holes in it to support the test tubes whilst testing urine. Then there were the Keto-Diastix tablets. Colour range from memory was a very pale colour to dark brown. If you urinated on a strip and it turned dark brown, you had no idea (really) how high your sugar levels were. You just had to trust your thirst level and of course your urine output, fatigue, and nausea.

So, when your dad invented the first blood machine for people with type1 diabetes. OMG!!!!!

It was the size of a brick, but it was such a breakthrough in the Diabetic World.

I remember it used to sit on my dressing table at home close to a power point. If the power went out so did the blood machine. It did however operate by battery also which was certainly a help when the power went out.

Next to my dressing table I had a basket with plastic in it, cos you had to wash the blood off the strip after a short period of time.

My dad still has my first blood machine your dad made.

A lot of my late mum's family lived in Bathurst. We often used to visit. I always remember. Mmmmmm, now where do I put this blood machine???? It needed to have its own safe place so I could monitor my glucose levels when I needed to.

Well, we have come a long, long way since then.

In some ways going through what we did Lisa makes us very aware now of the significance of what your dad did and created the path for the blood machines that are available today. I know you often say that a multi-national company came in and basically copied what your dad did. BUT he started the process, no matter what the legalities were that followed.

A very special man...STAN CLARK

Kind regards
**Leanne Eisenhuth**

What a difference that blood machine made. I remember meeting Stan and what a clever man! Inventing a machine to improve his daughter's diabetic life and as a result my daughters too. It gave us, Leanne's parents, great comfort that we understood her sugar levels more accurately. It was like a miracle and an absolute godsend. I still, to this day, have my daughters original blood machines.

With heartfelt memories and thanks.

**Laurie Shaw** *(Leanne Eisenhurth's father)*

I initially trained as an enrolled nurse between 1982-1984 and went on to qualify as a state registered nurse in 1991. It was during these early years in nursing that I developed my interest in diabetes as I worked on an acute medical ward (adult), that specialized in the condition. I recall using the old BM 1-44 testing strips on patients to assess their blood glucose levels. I also remember having to prick patients' fingers with the smallest needles that could be found from ward stocks, until specific finger lancets became more widely available. However, these early bloodletting procedures were often painful for patients with their poor fingers often left sore and excoriated from undergoing several finger pricks a day.

Sadly, during these years, I often saw the acute and long-term complications associated with diabetes, and the impact that this had on the lives of people living with the condition. My professional interest deepened because as complex and complicated as diabetes could be, it was a medical condition that could, with the right treatment, education, and tools, be self-managed by the patients themselves. This is why I undertook my first diabetes and teaching courses, which enabled me to take on the role of diabetes link nurse within the acute medical unit. In 1993 I was asked by our lead Diabetes Consultant if I would take up a Diabetes Specialist Nurse (DSN) post and join the existing two nurses who worked across the hospital and community setting. By this time, like so many other health districts across the UK, we were seeing many more people developing both types of diabetes and more complications. The need for greater investment in diabetes care was starting to gather pace. As the DSN role combined my two professional passions; education and diabetes, accepting it was a no brainer!

Between 1993 and 2003 I worked in the specialty of diabetes across two counties, Derbyshire, and Lincolnshire in both the acute and community settings. I remember vividly that on my first day in the Diabetes Unit at the Chesterfield Royal Hospital in Derbyshire, the senior diabetes nurse showed me her archive of old 'brick' sized meters. In her dual role as pediatric and adult diabetes nurse, she had once upon a time used them. The first meter I recall using was a Reflolux S, small in comparison to its predecessors but of course, now a dinosaur! Meter technology continued to move at a rapid pace particularly in terms of size and design. Lancet and lancet devices were also becoming much less vicious when pricking the finger and test strips required much smaller amounts of blood. I cannot count the number of patients I saw who stated that learning how to test their blood glucose levels and having access to portable monitoring equipment was absolutely life changing for them. I recall one lady who had had diabetes for over 40 years. She showed me the very first portable glucose meter that she had used as an 11-year-old child and said that it saved her life. Although she had upgraded long before our first meeting, she was attached to her 'life saver' and would not part with it even for our archive collection!

The impact of diabetes on those living with it fascinated me such that in 1999, I based the dissertation for my first degree in professional nursing practice, on the physiological and psychosocial well-being of people with diabetes. By this time, I had worked for several years within the specialty, in both a clinical and educational role. I can categorically state that the confidence that patients gained when being able to undertake home blood glucose monitoring was immense, particularly when adjusting insulin treatments and managing sick days. From a professional perspective it was an absolute joy to see technology make life easier and safer for patients. Unfortunately, I also remember that many of our GPs (General Practitioners), would refuse to re-prescribe blood glucose test strips and actively encouraged patients to cut test strips in half! Although times have thankfully changed, during these earlier years some practitioners were more concerned about savings in the short term to their practice budgets, rather than the longer-term benefits to their diabetes patients and the NHS!

In 2003 I became the first Nurse Consultant for Diabetes in Derbyshire. This unique role enabled me to champion further the case for proper investment in diabetes care, not just at a local and regional level, but also on a national stage. I was also able to develop and expand my own and my teams clinical and educational practices further. By this time there was an increasing body of research evidence and Department of Health (DoH) documents, that identified that quality diabetes services, to include patient education and access to self-management tools could improve diabetes outcomes significantly. Following the successful outcomes of the DAFNE insulin skills training program, my team and I developed our own local patient education course - A Skills Program in matching Insulin Requirements to Eating and exercise (ASPIRE) in 2005. I thought the acronym appropriate given our aims and objectives and also because we have a famous crooked spire in Chesterfield! The course proved to be very successful with our Type 1 students and was used for the basis of my master's research in Diabetes in 2007, with outcomes on the small study published in 2008.

In my experience and professional opinion, the development of the original blood glucose meter into a portable device that could be used by patients at home was an absolute game changer in the management of diabetes. The undertaking of self-blood glucose monitoring in the home/social and work settings has been pivotal in not only providing evidence about improved blood glucose parameters but in significantly reducing hospital admissions and diabetes related complications. Furthermore, all of the successful insulin skills programs during my specialty years required multiple blood glucose monitoring to be undertaken by all Type 1 students who wanted to access such a course. Over many years I also saw the confidence, freedom and sense of security that being able to blood glucose monitor brought to people with diabetes enabling them to take control of their condition and lead a 'normal' life.

To find out in recent times, that Uncle Stan was a fore father of this technology has been wonderful and I have read with great interest his story. The fact that he developed his portable blood glucose monitoring equipment purely for altruistic reasons and not commercial gain, makes him a hero in my opinion. A sentiment that I am sure would be shared by anyone involved in the international diabetes community who learns about his work.

**Dee Clark**

My daughter, Lilly, was first diagnosed with type 1 diabetes in 2008 when she was 2 years old. The hospital gave us a small portable blood glucose monitor when she was first diagnosed, and we left the hospital to go home to try and deal with the horrible illness on our own. I took it for granted that we could take this small machine with us anywhere and everywhere we went. Being so young and small, her blood sugars were very volatile and would be up and down for no known reason. There was no stability and no pattern. We had no clue whether her blood glucose levels were 1.6 or 33.3 or anything in-between. She showed only the mildest of symptoms at either extreme.

At first, we would check her blood sugars fairy regularly, before meals, after meals, before we went out, before bedtime, during the night. We would check before we left the house and then do whatever we had on that day. I still vividly remember one day, early on in her diagnosis, we went for a walk to the shops which were about a 5-minute walk away from our house. We didn't take the blood glucose monitor because we were just going up the street. Suddenly, I could see all the colour drain from her face and my usual very active little girl had gone all limp. Low blood sugars I guessed. But were they low or were they high?? I didn't know. So, I treated Lilly, assuming she was low by giving her lollies to eat, hoping her blood sugars weren't actually high, and I wasn't actually making high blood sugars even higher and Lilly even sicker. From that day on I never left the house without a blood glucose monitor. Thanks to Stanley Clark we had the ability to always have a meter with us, so we could check and know for sure what her blood sugar levels really were.

Years later I met another type 1 diabetic who was in her 40's. She would tell me horror stories of when her mother used to have to use urine strips to check her blood sugars which was such an inaccurate way of checking them. Her Mum also used to have to boil something up on the stove again to check blood sugars. Again, only an indication of what the blood sugars were hours before. Having to do this would have made looking after your young child's diabetes near impossible. I remember thinking at the time 'thank goodness we are living with diabetes in this time, and not before when it was a huge effort just to do a test that we can complete in near seconds these days.

We were so lucky to have an instant accurate reading of her blood sugars in real time. Lilly has always maintained a Hb1AC in the target range and I credit this to the fact that she has had a blood glucose monitor on hand to continuously check her blood sugars. Lilly has also never been so hypoglycaemic that she has passed out, we have caught all the lows on the meter often before she showed any symptoms at all. Conversely all her highs were caught on the meter so we could take immediate action to bring her blood sugars down.

In 2017 when Lilly was in year 6, she completed a 'Night of Notables' project. This project entailed picking someone who had made a notable contribution to society, researching them, and putting together a story board of their achievements. We had seen earlier that Stanley Clark had invented the first portable blood meter in Australia back in the 1970's. Lilly decided to try and contact Lisa, Stanley's daughter as we had heard that Stanley had sadly passed away. Lilly made contact with Lisa and then a little later with Stanley's wife Audrey, who was an integral part of the development and commercialisation of the world's first portable blood glucose meter. We were blown away with just how generous, kind, friendly and loving these two women are. They spent hours with us giving us information, pictures, photos, and the actual prototype of the meter that Stanley had made. They shared all their stories and gave us such a detailed insight into what they went through when Lisa was a small child battling with her diabetes.

Stanley and Audrey's desperate love for their daughter lead to the invention of the world's first potable blood glucose meter, purely so they could better care for their daughter and by doing this all the other parents struggling with their diabetic children, could do the same.

Lilly had to find a quote from her Night of Notable to use in her project, she picked a quote of Stanley's own words, which encompasses exactly what the Clark's were about, "It's been designed for people, not for money". Stanley and Audrey had one goal, that was to help not only their daughter, but all the diabetic children and adults wherever they were in the world to better care for themselves and not have to run continuously backwards and forwards to hospital.

**Viv Todd**

Hi Lisa, wow. Lovely to meet you.

I was diagnosed in 1967 at the age of 2.
I was introduced to the BSL machine when I was 15. My memory may not be one that you put in your book though. Lol. Here it is.
My mother took me to the clinic at the RNSH in a place they called "The cottage". They took us in and showed the machine. Then told me to put out my hand and poked a lancet in it. Perhaps if I was forewarned it might have been different.

We walked out of the cottage, and I told my mother. "I won't ever use that."

Lol to think of it now.

Of course, we took one home, and it sat around for quite a while. But I must have relented as I then used it off and on through my teenage years but got serious about looking after the diabetes more when I reached my twenties so used it constantly. Even 10 times a day during my pregnancies.

Now I am on CGM and the pump and I say that I blood tested for 35 years.

I'm a disability carer and have two children a boy 28 and a girl 30. Neither with diabetes.

**Cheers Cathy Hickey**

Hi Lisa,

I can only say thank you for the chance to say thanks to your family and especially your dad. I've read about his life in an article from the Sydney Morning Herald and he must have been very special to make a meter for you. The Stanley Clark glucose meter was a life changer for me. I moved to Chatswood in 1985 and heard about your dad's meter in a magazine. I drove over to Dee Why and bought the machine straight from the front door. It was pretty expensive for me at the time, about $100 but well worth every cent. I never realised until tonight reading an article about your dad how generous he was selling his meters at cost. Beforehand, I used the Clinistix urine strips that were known to be very unreliable. Like yourself, at the time, the only other blood test was at the hospital.

Kind regards,
**Michael Ginges**

I was diagnosed with Diabetes Mellitus Type 1 in 1983 I was 18 years old, living in England.

It was a shock to my system physically though more so mentally. I could not get my head around needles for one and the thought of no longer being able to be free to do whatever I wanted to do when it came to eating, partying, playing sport and dancing (I was in my prime). How was I going to go out drinking and dancing? How would I be able to control my blood sugar levels when I only knew the levels by going to the hospital outpatient's department on a regular basis. I could always test my urine with the strips, but this was never reliable and non-consistent with the way I was feeling. I really was not in control of the diabetes it controlled everything about me.

In 1985 I was able to loan a machine from the diabetic clinic, which was huge, bulky, and very heavy. I had to carry this around like a large heavy handbag though despite this I was delighted with not having to go daily to the hospital for a testing.

For my birthday in 1986 my family put their money together and purchased a home glucose meter for me. This was a much smaller compact blood sugar testing machine it cost them over 120 pounds and was the greatest birthday present I had ever received. I will always be grateful for this gift which gave me more freedom and more control.

I have recently been searching for the history of different ways of checking blood sugar levels, it was in the 1980's when self-monitoring blood sugars at home became more common (and was I glad about this) it certainly changed my life, and I began to take control of my diabetes for once. I became confident and no longer afraid all the time of hypo/hyper episodes.

Stanley Clark inventor of the battery-operated blood glucose monitor for whom I am forever grateful gave millions of people the confidence to be in control of diabetes and to live life which did not involve daily trips to the hospital for testing.

I am now 55 years old living in Australia I work as a care facilitator for elderly people, and I am honoured to be care facilitator for Stanley Clark's beautiful wife Audrey and close friend to his fabulous daughter Lisa. There is no better way I can repay Stanley for the freedom he gave to me personally with a home monitoring glucose machine than to assist in the care of his wonderful wife Audrey.

**Sue Bailey**

My Uncle Stan

Uncle Stan was my mother's youngest brother. My mother, Ada, absolutely adored my Uncle Stan.

Sadly, both my mother and Uncle Stan died of Alzheimers.

I clearly remember visions of uncle Stan's lovely smile, his sincerity, his love of "Mother Nature" and his many references to her! His genuine interest and compassion for people who'd been special in his life and just even his desire to look up people that he'd known as he wanted to find out how they were getting on whilst he was in the country. I loved that he took me with him to meet these people. I don't think I realised why then, as a child, just that I loved him taking me to meet 'his people' as I saw it then! He was such a gentle man, kind, and thoughtful and I was always so excited when Mum said that Aunt Audrey and Uncle Stan were planning on coming for a holiday. You may think this as funny as me, but when Aunt Audrey and Uncle Stan went off to Australia to live, I remembered them saying to me they'd send me a koala bear. I waited and waited for said koala bear. (I was 5!) I can picture in my mind, Mum coming into my bedroom one morning sometime after they'd gone, switching the light on in the dark morning and saying I'd got a parcel from Australia! Uncle Stan and Aunt Audrey! I was so disappointed because when I opened the parcel it WAS a koala bear.... But it wasn't a real one!   At 5 years old that was such a big disappointment! I really had thought they'd send me a REAL koala! Hilarious, but it's true!

My Husband and two sons think he was special too and I'm so very grateful that they have memories of him.

He was just the most iconic " uncle" *for me, but for the rest of my family who only knew him a brief time, he was also loved for the person he was... Special... MY UNCLE STAN XX

We hold the special people in our hearts forever, Uncle Stan was and will always be special to all of us.

In the meantime, so is Aunt Audrey.  She is THE most special Auntie / great Auntie.

**Linda Payne**


Hi Lisa

I attended a Diabetes education program at the cottage at Royal North Shore Hospital back in the day and I remember you and your mum being on the same education program.  It would have been either late 1977 or early 1978.  I was 15 and you would have been around 10 at the time.  I remember sometime after that your dad building one of those glucose testers and I was lucky enough to get hold of one. I think it was lent to me by either the Cottage at Royal North Shore Hospital or my specialist at the time.  I remember it being the size of a small house brick and it involved some lens cleaning.

I will be forever grateful to your dad for the perseverance he showed in getting the prototype off the ground so it could evolve into the technology we have today.

**Carmel Howard**

If memory serves me correctly, I believe I first met Stan as a work colleague when he joined Hanimex. I had moved from Melbourne to take a position as a junior design engineer at Hanimex some 10 years earlier.

Hanimex at that time was a very large importer, distributor and manufacturer of home photographic equipment and accessories based at Brookvale, a Sydney northern beaches suburb. Manufactured products included slide projectors, movie projectors, slide viewers, a range of table lamps and room heaters and reel-to-reel tape recorders. All were designed by Hanimex staff and all the manufacturing operations were carried out within the Brookvale facility, a totally vertically integrated operation with almost individual components for the products produced "in-house".

In the mid-seventies we had just begun the manufacture of a home entertainment centre, an ensemble that included a radio, a record player, and a cassette player. The manufacturing team soon realized that they needed more technical support on the assembly floor, especially from someone with electronic engineering skills and experience – hence Stan's appointment.

Stan made a big difference. He was able to quickly identify problems and suggest improvements and that brought him into contact with the design team. It didn't take us long to realize that here was someone who could make a difference and not just with our electronic products but across the entire manufactured product range. From then on Stan was invited to participate in the design process by assisting with prototype building and testing. Throughout this process Stan and I worked closely together and as well as being work colleagues we became good friends.

I often visited Stan at home to see the latest projects he was working on in his well-equipped workshop and here I was introduced to his wife Audrey and daughter Lisa, both very supportive of Stan and very much part of the Stan Clark enterprise. It was during these visits that I found out quite a lot more about Stan and how he developed his creative skills.

I learned that Stan was born and schooled in the UK, I think Sheffield. As a young lad he was, inquisitive, enquiring and determined to find out "what made things tick", and encouraged by his father in these endeavours. A well-equipped home workshop was at his disposal, and it was here that he developed his skills in experimenting and making things. As he became older his knowledge, skills and experience developed; he became a licensed amateur (ham) radio operator and a qualified motor vehicle mechanic. One of Stan's major achievements at this time was the design and manufacture of a portable TV receiver in the UK, a unique achievement that attracted quite a lot of attention from the press – as he showed me as we became better acquainted. Stan was justifiably proud of his achievements but never one to boast about them.

At about this time the UK had a compulsory National Service scheme requiring physically fit males within the ages of 17 to 24 years to serve a period of 18 months (this was later extended to 2 years) with one of the armed services. Stan chose the Royal Air Force, and it didn't take them long to put his knowledge of electronics and radio communication to use. He was appointed as the "technical skills" member of a small surveillance team planted somewhere in Europe (he never disclosed where) to intercept soviet military radio traffic. His role was to make sure that their equipment was always in first class operating condition. Although he endured a few hardships, the freezing cold months of winter being one, he did enjoy it and has many interesting stories from this time with me.

It was during one of our discussions at Hanimex, probably in the Canteen over lunch, that Stan mentioned his interest in developing a blood glucose monitor to be used by diabetics. I learned that Stan's daughter was diabetic and that for her, like all diabetes sufferers, diet and medication needed to be closely controlled to maintain blood glucose levels within defined limits. In those days expensive instruments were used to measure blood glucose concentrations, instruments that were usually only found in hospitals and specialist clinics. Home monitoring usually involved careful observation of symptoms and sometimes urine testing with reagent tablets – the instruments used in the hospitals and clinics were beyond the means of most families. Stan was aware of this and resolved to do something about it.

Working with one of the medical specialists responsible for treating diabetic children at the Children's Hospital Stan gained an understanding of the operating principles of blood glucose measuring devices used in the hospital environment and had soon built a prototype that could do the same job as the instruments in the hospital but at a very much reduced cost. More protypes were produced and given to families to use at home to monitor their children's blood glucose levels. These trials soon confirmed that Stan's device was just as effective as those used in the hospital and that it could be manufactured at a cost that was within the means of most households and in other cases, with support from diabetes charities, offered to families free-of-charge.

The demand for Stan's blood glucose monitoring device grew so rapidly that he could no longer keep up demand and still work for Hanimex – this was his life's work and he needed to devote all of his time to it. I still kept in touch and found that he had moved his operation from home to rented premises beneath a fish shop in Dee Why, a Sydney northern beaches suburb. It was not long after this move that Stan called to tell me that was planning to introduce a new model incorporating enhanced features and a design to suit large scale manufacturing and assembly methods – similar to those he had seen at Hanimex. I was only too happy to advise on the design of components that could be manufactured using plastic injection moulding processes and to recommend an engineer who could specify and program a microprocessor that would now be at the heart of the instrument. This new device and the planned increase in output required Stan to relinquish the Dee Why address, it was way too small, and move a little south to Brookvale where he found a large industrial unit.

Stan became very busy manufacturing his new device and developing new markets for it. I didn't see him often at this time but when we did catch up, I found he had not only increased his local market but was in the advanced stages of developing export markets.

One new project Stan was working on at the time, was the development of the reagent strip that was part of the blood glucose monitoring system. The strip was a small narrow paper strip with a reagent chemical located at its tip. To make the blood glucose measurement the thumb is pricked with fine needle raising a small drop of blood. This drop is transferred to the reagent tip of the strip which causes it to change colour, the hue being dependent on the glucose concentration in the blood. This end of the strip is then inserted into the measuring instrument which measures the colour and reports the corresponding blood glucose concentration. Stan worked in collaboration with a university professor of chemistry on this development.

Word of Stan's development of the reagent strip soon got around and especially to one large US manufacturer of blood glucose monitoring equipment. This company was aware of the instrument Stan had put on the market and presumably did not see it as a big threat to their sales however they saw the supply of an opposition reagent strip as a big threat. Each customer only needs one monitoring instrument, but they need hundreds and hundreds of reagent strips per year and that is where they make most of their money – Stan now represented a big threat to their business, and they were determined to put him out of business. They undercut prices in every market that Stan operated in and kept that up until he could no longer sustain his losses forcing him to shut down his operation.

I did see Stan from time to time after this period and found that he had a new interest, a housing property development project in the northern part of NSW but I think he missed the product development that gave him so much satisfaction.

I had also move on eventually finding myself at ResCare (later to be renamed ResMed), a very new company that had developed a device for treating obstructive sleep apnoea. ResMed had two quite small product engineering development teams at that time, one electrical and one mechanical, I was the manager of the mechanical engineering team.

With ResCare's rapid growth it soon became obvious that we needed more help in the building of engineering prototypes and we advertised such a position. In amongst a large number of applications was one from Stan Clark and it was immediately obvious that it was from the Stan Clark and that he was the ideal candidate - Stan was appointed. Not only did he help with the building of our prototypes but in the process, he often made very helpful suggestions on how they might be improved, as I knew he would from my Hanimex experience.

Stan was with us for quite a few years until he and his wife Audrey, who also worked at, by now, ResMed, in the account's office, decided to sell up in Sydney and retire to a more northerly location in NSW. I didn't see much of him after that, but I knew that he had moved his home-workshop and all of its equipment with him, so I imagine that he spent a lot of his time inventing and making all sorts of interesting devices.

Apart from his creative flair another thing I discovered about Stan was the strength of his hands, it was formidable. At ResMed he was responsible for our small prototype building workshop within which there were a large number of screw-cap containers for all sorts of components. The contents of these containers were inaccessible to the rest of us if Stan had been there before – we couldn't get the caps off. We had to continually remind him to be extra gentle. Heaven knows how Audrey and Lisa got on at home with screw-cap containers in the kitchen, no sauce or jam or pickles in the Clark household.

**Bob Styles.**

My name is Nick Warry and I have been a type 1 diabetic since 1994 when I was 11 years old. Having this disease for almost three decades now, I have experienced the many advancements in technology and medicine surrounding the management of diabetes with testing and insulin. In particular, mobile blood glucose level (BGL) testing has been a literal life saver. Upon first being diagnosed with diabetes, portable BGL testers used to take up to 60 seconds to give a result and required double the amount of blood when compared to the BGL machines today, which can give a result in as little as 5 seconds. Throughout my many years as a diabetic, I have always been fortunate enough to have excellent control of my BGLs. This has only been possible with constant testing with a glucose meter. On average I normally test at least 10 times a day so that I can adjust my insulin levels to match what my body is doing. A very big misconception with diabetes is that food is the only thing that will affect BGL. This is definitely not true at all. Everything can have an effect on BGL, such as: • not getting enough sleep (BGL goes low/high) • stress (BGL goes high) • sunburn (BGL goes high) • exercising below your fitness level (BGL goes low slowly) • exercising above your fitness level (BGL goes high then low) • high Glycemic Index (GI) foods (BGL goes high quickly) • low GI foods (BGL goes high slowly) • fatty/oily foods (BGL goes low and then high) • caffeine (BGL goes low) • climbing a ladder (BGL goes low – every time I even look at one) As can be seen above the list is expansive and this is a highly summarised version, the list is also endless. Coupled with this list is also the fact that everybody has a different body and so will have a different BGL response to different things. This makes managing diabetes without testing a bit harder than juggling four live snakes and two cats at the same time blindfolded... with one hand tied behind your back... in short it would be next to impossible. The long-term effects of bad BGL management can include blindness, amputations or even death. Fortunately, having the ability to have accurate and portable BGL testing makes living with diabetes possible. I have been able to work, travel, exercise, relax and live life the same way someone without diabetes does, just with constant testing and insulin management. I now have a continuous BGL monitor attached to my arm giving me even more control than before, so I look forward to what the future technologies and advancements in medicine bring. None of this though would be possible without the creation of a portable BGL tester. I know without this, as a diabetic, I would not have had the same quality of life or may not be living today, and so because of this I cannot express enough my thanks and gratitude to the pioneering inventor and engineer Stanley Clark who made it possible. Proving that necessity is the mother (or in this case "daughter" – Lisa Harris nee Clark) of all invention.